D0533836

DIABETES

HARTLEP... BOROUGH
WITHDRAWN
LIB...RIES

1434775 X

Published in 2007 by Murdoch Books Pty Limited
www.murdochbooks.com.au

Murdoch Books Australia
Pier 8/9
23 Hickson Road
Millers Point NSW 2000
Phone: +61 (0) 2 8220 2000
Fax: +61 (0) 2 8220 2558

Murdoch Books UK Limited
Erico House
6th Floor
93–99 Upper Richmond Road
Putney, London SW15 2TG
Phone: +44 (0) 20 8785 5995
Fax: +44 (0) 20 8785 5985

Chief Executive: Juliet Rogers
Publishing Director: Kay Scarlett

Design manager: Vivien Valk
Project manager and editor: Emma Hutchinson
Recipe consultant and nutrition analyst: Susanna Holt
Design concept: Susanne Geppert
Designer: Anthony Vandenberg
Photographer: Ian Hofstetter
Stylists: Jane Collins and Katy Holder
Food preparation: Joanne Kelly and Grace Campbell
Recipes by: Michelle Earl and members of the Murdoch Books Test Kitchen
Production: Maiya Levitch

Text, design and photography copyright Murdoch Books 2007. All rights reserved. No part of this publication may be reproduced, stored in a retrieval system or transmitted in any form or by any means, electronic, mechanical, photocopying, recording or otherwise, without the prior written permission of the publisher.

National Library of Australia Cataloguing-in-Publication Data

Kingham, Karen.
Eat well live well with -- diabetes : low GI recipes and tips.

Includes index.
ISBN 978 1 74045 962 4 (pbk.).

1. Diabetes - Diet therapy. 2. Glycemic index. 3. Food - Carbohydrate content. I. Title.

613.283

Printed by Sing Cheong Printing Co. Ltd. in 2007. PRINTED IN HONG KONG.
Reprinted 2007 (twice), 2008 (twice).

The Publisher and stylist would like to thank Dinosaur Designs, Mud Australia, Bison Homewares and IKEA for assistance in the photography of this book.

IMPORTANT: Those who might be at risk from the effects of salmonella poisoning (the elderly, pregnant women, young children and those suffering from immune deficiency diseases) should consult their doctor with any concerns about eating raw eggs.

CONVERSION GUIDE: You may find cooking times vary depending on the oven you are using. For fan-forced ovens, as a general rule, set the oven temperature to 20°C (35°F) lower than indicated in the recipe. We have used 20 ml (4 teaspoon) tablespoon measures. If you are using a 15 ml (3 teaspoon) tablespoon, for most recipes the difference will not be noticeable. However, for recipes using baking powder, gelatine, bicarbonate of soda (baking soda), small amounts of flour and cornflour (cornstarch), add an extra teaspoon for each tablespoon specified.

EATWELLLIVEWELL
with DIABETES
Low-GI recipes and tips

Introductory text by Karen Kingham (nutritionist)

HARTLEPOOL BOROUGH LIBRARIES	
1434775X	
Bertrams	20/10/2008
641.563	£9.99
HO	

MURDOCH BOOKS

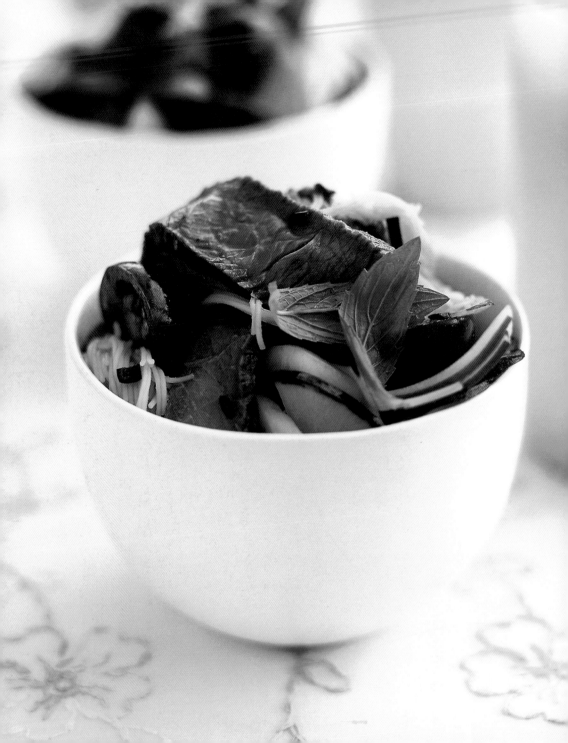

CONTENTS

LIVING WITH DIABETES

Diabetes affects more than 230 million people worldwide and is one of the fastest growing diseases in the world. Because the risk of developing diabetes is influenced by lifestyle, there are steps you can take to reduce this risk, control it once you've been diagnosed or even reverse some of its unwanted effects.

In the past, people with diabetes followed rigid diet plans with little room for enjoyment. Today, thanks to good scientific research, diet and lifestyle recommendations for diabetes differ very little from those made for everyone else; a healthy diet balanced for your individual needs, plus daily exercise.

You may also be pleasantly surprised to learn that healthy food can be, and is delicious if you know how to prepare it. And, once you get to the end of this book you will be convinced of it.

Who will benefit from this book?

If you have diabetes or are at risk of developing it, or you care for someone who has it, then you will find this book useful. Diabetes doesn't have to mean separate meals or eating differently to everyone else. All the recipes in this book can be enjoyed by family and friends alike, which is especially important when children have diabetes. No child wants to be different, and in many ways their diet doesn't have to be. The recipes in this book will help them—or any one else for that matter—achieve a healthy, balanced diet.

What is diabetes?

Diabetes results in a build-up of sugar (known as glucose) in the bloodstream. This happens when the body can't make enough of the hormone insulin, or is unable to use insulin properly.

To understand why and how this happens you need to understand a little about how the body works. The level of glucose in the blood rises whenever you eat any carbohydrate (sugars or starches). As the carbohydrate is digested, glucose is absorbed into the bloodstream. As the blood glucose level rises, it stimulates the pancreas to release the hormone insulin. The insulin enables the body's cells to absorb the glucose from the blood, so that the cells can use it for energy (or store it to use as energy later on).

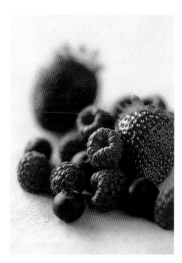

Insulin works much like a key that fits a lock to open the door to the cells. Without insulin, glucose remains trapped within the blood. The action of insulin, in concert with other hormones, keeps you blood glucose level steady.

Diabetes develops when the pancreas either doesn't make enough insulin or the body becomes resistant to the effects of insulin. In both cases, the result is that glucose is unable to get to the cells and builds up in the bloodstream.

Over time, a high blood glucose level can damage the eyes, nerves and blood vessels as well as increase the risk of heart disease, kidney and circulation problems. Early diagnosis and good blood glucose control are essential in preventing these serious health problems.

There are several different types of diabetes and they all result in too much glucose in the bloodstream:

Type 1 diabetes

Sometimes called insulin-dependent diabetes or juvenile-onset diabetes, type 1 diabetes is the least common but the most serious form of diabetes. It typically begins in childhood or early adulthood, but can occur at any age.

Type 1 diabetes is an autoimmune disease in which the body's immune system destroys cells in the pancreas that are responsible for making insulin. Scientists believe that exposure to a particular virus or chemical may trigger this immune reaction in susceptible people.

Ultimately, the pancreas stops making insulin and the blood glucose level rises dramatically. The symptoms that result include excessive thirst, frequent urination, blurred vision, abdominal cramps and nausea.

Weight loss is also very common as the body burns up fat and muscle tissue to use as energy instead of blood glucose. Symptoms will usually appear very suddenly

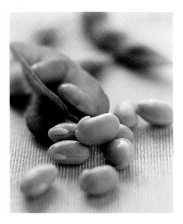

due to the speed with which glucose builds up in the blood once insulin production fails.

Unlike the other forms of diabetes, excess weight is not the reason for the development of type 1 diabetes, and most people are a healthy weight at the time their diabetes begins.

Blood glucose levels in type 1 diabetes are managed with regular daily insulin injections, healthy eating and an active lifestyle.

Type 2 diabetes

Also known as non-insulin dependent diabetes or adult onset diabetes, this type of diabetes is the most common, affecting up to 90 per cent of all people with diabetes.

Type 2 diabetes is largely found in people over 40 years of age who are overweight and have a family history of diabetes. However, recently type 2 diabetes is being seen in younger adults and even children, due to our population becoming less active and more overweight.

In type 2 diabetes the pancreas continues to make insulin (unlike type 1 diabetes) but the body doesn't respond to it as well and becomes resistant to its effects. This is known as insulin resistance. The pancreas makes more insulin to compensate, but over time this still isn't enough. Eventually the blood glucose level remains elevated.

The onset of type 2 diabetes is typically a gradual process, unlike type 1 diabetes. In fact, many people with type 2 diabetes won't have any noticeable symptoms early on, and so won't be aware they have the condition. Once blood glucose begins to rise significantly, the following symptoms may be experienced: excessive thirst, frequent urination, blurred vision, thrush, more frequent infections, poor wound healing and fatigue.

Type 2 diabetes can often be managed with healthy eating, an active lifestyle and weight loss alone. The best way to achieve this will be different for every individual, so it is important to follow the advice of a doctor, dietitian or diabetes educator. In addition to losing weight with healthy diet and exercise, some people with type 2 diabetes might also need medication. This may be tablets that help reduce insulin resistance and in some cases insulin injections as well.

Risk factors for type 2 diabetes?

If you have one or more of the following factors, then you are at risk of type 2 diabetes and should visit your doctor as soon as possible.

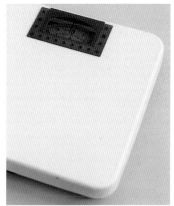

- I am over 45 years old and overweight
- I am over 45 years old and have high blood pressure
- I am over 45 years old and do very little physical activity
- I am over 45 years old and have one or more family members with diabetes
- I am over 35 years old and am of Asian, Southern European, Indian, Hispanic, Aboriginal, Torres Strait Islander or Polynesian descent
- I am over 55 years old
- I have had a heart attack or stroke
- I have had gestational diabetes or my baby weighed over 4 kg (8 lb 12 oz) at birth
- I am overweight and have polycystic ovarian syndrome (PCOS)
- I am overweight, with most of my weight around my middle rather than on my hips and thighs
- I have high blood pressure, a high blood cholesterol or high triglyceride level

Gestational diabetes

Gestational diabetes is a type of diabetes, usually temporary, that develops during pregnancy, around the second or third trimester. Insulin needs are higher in pregnancy and the hormones produced during this time can reduce the effectiveness of insulin. It is diagnosed by a blood test at around 24 to 28 weeks gestation and is similar to type 2 diabetes where the body is resistant to the effects of insulin.

It is estimated that between 3 and 8 per cent of pregnant women can't meet their body's extra demands for insulin and end up with gestational diabetes. Women at greatest risk are those over 30 years of age with a family history of type 2 diabetes and those who are overweight. Other risk factors include being of Chinese, Indian or Aboriginal descent or previously having had a baby weighing more than 4 kg (8 lb 12 oz).

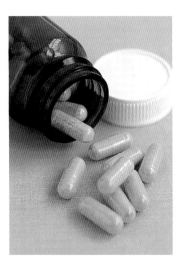

Gestational diabetes is controlled with a healthy diet, an active lifestyle and strict monitoring of blood glucose levels. If this isn't enough to keep blood glucose levels in check then insulin injections are needed and some women may need to be admitted to hospital. Well-managed blood glucose levels are important to your health and the baby's. Poorly controlled blood glucose levels cause your baby to grow bigger and fatter. This makes delivery more difficult and increases the risk of complications such as miscarriage and health problems for the baby.

Gestational diabetes usually goes away once the baby is born but it does increase the risk for developing type 2 diabetes later in life for both you and your child. These risks can be reduced by maintaining a healthy weight, eating a healthy diet and staying active.

Pre-diabetes

Pre-diabetes occurs when blood glucose levels are higher than normal but not high enough to be diagnosed as diabetes. It is also known as Impaired Glucose Tolerance (IGT) or Impaired Fasting Glucose (IFG).

Like type 2 diabetes, pre-diabetes is due to the body becoming resistant to the effects of insulin. The risk of pre-diabetes becoming type 2 diabetes is high. However, research shows that you can reverse this risk simply by improving your diet and lifestyle. This means controlling your weight, losing weight if you are carrying excess, reducing the amount of fat you eat, increasing your fibre intake, switching to low glycaemic index carbohydrates and being more active—aiming for at least 30 minutes of exercise a day, or more if you need to lose weight. In fact, research shows that these strategies can be even more effective than medication in reversing the progress of pre-diabetes toward type 2 diabetes.

How common is diabetes?

The International Diabetes Federation estimates that six million people worldwide develop diabetes each year, and that in some countries as many as 80 per cent of these people won't know it. They also predict that by 2025, diabetes will affect 350 million people, which is equivalent to a serious worldwide diabetes epidemic.

Why is diabetes on the increase? The most important factor is the ever-expanding weight of the world's population. The rise in diabetes is closely coupled to rising rates of obesity. In some countries obesity rates have more than tripled in the last 20 years, and there are now around 1.3 billion overweight people in the world—which outnumbers the world's starving. It is little wonder then that the chronic illnesses brought on by overweight and obesity—like type 2 diabetes—are also on the rise.

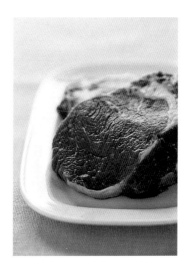

In many ways the statistics are more alarming for those who are not yet diagnosed. Being unaware of your diabetes puts you at greater risk of health complications from chronically high blood glucose levels. For this reason everyone at risk of diabetes (see page 10) should make it a priority to have regular check-ups with their doctor.

What health problems can be caused by diabetes?

Damage to the body occurs when blood glucose levels are chronically high. Over time this may result in permanent damage to your blood vessels and the tissues or organs they supply. In the case of type 2 diabetes this may have been happening for some time before you even know about it. In many cases, the complications of high blood glucose levels (nerve problems, heart attack, vision disturbances) lead to a diagnosis of type 2 diabetes.

Once you have been diagnosed with diabetes, keeping your blood glucose level within the normal range, or as close to the normal range as possible, is vital. By doing this you can prevent or slow the onset of the serious health complications associated with diabetes. The most common complications include:

Cardiovascular disease

People with diabetes are around five times more likely to develop heart disease and can be up to four times more likely to suffer a stroke than those without diabetes.

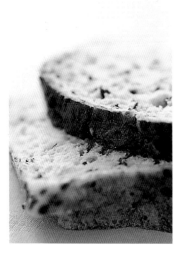

Damage to blood vessels caused by diabetes also affects the circulation, particularly in the legs. This poor circulation makes cuts and infections slow to heal. A diet low in saturated fat and high in fibre with antioxidant-rich vegetables and fruit is essential when you have diabetes for reducing your risk of cardiovascular desease.

Nerve damage

Also known as neuropathy, nerve damage results in the loss of sensation and/or pain in the hands and feet as well as problems with the functioning of many of the body's systems.

One of the complications of nerve damage, especially affecting the legs and feet, occurs when numbness allows injuries to go unnoticed. People with diabetes should have regular foot check-ups for this reason.

Kidney disease

Kidney disease can occur when the blood vessels of the kidney are damaged by high blood glucose. Diabetes is a leading cause of kidney failure and people with diabetes are four times more likely to develop kidney disease than someone without diabetes.

Eye diseases

Diabetic retinopathy, a disease affecting the blood vessels of the retina, is the most common eye-related complication of diabetes. Keeping eye problems at bay can be helped by having regular check-ups with your ophthalmologist (eye specialist) or optometrist. A diet rich in vegetables and fruits will also help as antioxidants help protect the delicate blood vessels in eyes.

Living well with diabetes

Taking control of your diabetes means having the knowledge and support to make the best choices about your health and lifestyle. Access to health professionals such as your doctor, diabetes specialist physician, dietitian, diabetes educator, podiatrist and ophthalmologist (eye specialist) will mean the changes you make will be based on accurate up-to-date medical information. It is important to follow-up with your health team regularly to make sure that your blood glucose remains sufficiently under control.

Joining your local diabetes support group will also offer enormous benefits in terms of advice, support, reduced price products and many other services.

Why change your diet and lifestyle?

The main goal for anyone with diabetes is to keep their blood glucose level within the normal range and minimize long-term health problems. To do this, the right food in the right amounts plus regular exercise and weight control is essential. If you are overweight, a weight loss of as little as 5 per cent will help improve our blood glucose control, which will help reduce your risk of developing the complications of diabetes.

> **Dietary goals for people with diabetes**
> - less fat, especially the saturated kind
> - choose low glycaemic index (GI) and wholegrain carbohydrate foods
> - choose lean meat, chicken, fish and their alternatives such as nuts and seeds
> - use low-fat dairy foods or their alternatives
> - eat only modest amounts of sugar and sugar-containing foods
> - use less salt
> - only drink alcohol in moderation if at all

Tips for eating a healthy balanced diet when you have diabetes

What is healthy eating for diabetes?

Diabetes is a health problem that is greatly affected by the amount and types of food you eat. Therefore, a healthy diet is an essential part of its management. Advances in science mean there is now no such thing as a 'diabetic' diet or one specific diet that suits everyone with diabetes. In fact, healthy eating guidelines recommended for the whole population also apply to people with diabetes.

Because everyone with diabetes is different, the finer points of these recommendations will vary from person to person. It is a good idea to take on the challenge of overhauling your diet with the guidance of a dietitian. A dietitian will ensure any advice is tailored to your individual needs and that, where possible, the foods you enjoy are still included in your diet plan.

Watch your fat intake, especially saturated fat

Too much fat won't help with weight control, and if you have diabetes the chances are you need to lose weight. Too much saturated and trans fat will also worsen insulin

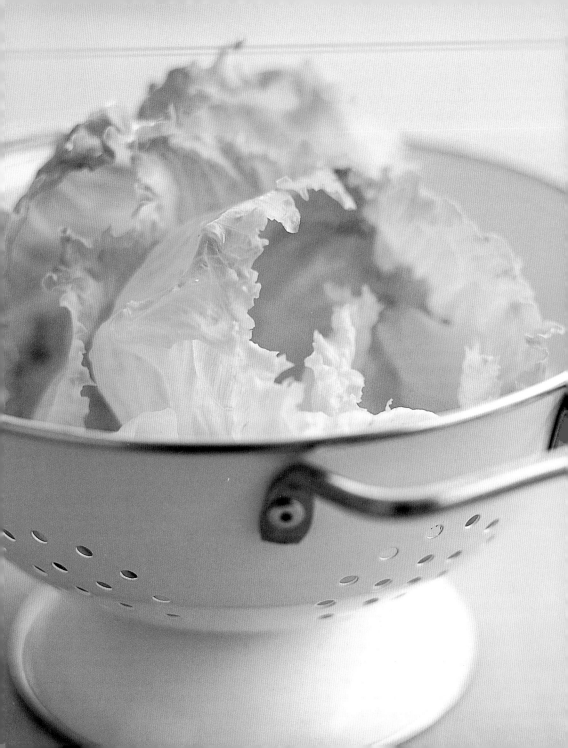

What fat is that?

Fat	Where will you find it?
Saturated fats	butter, cream, palm oil, coconut milk and cream, fried foods and takeaways, fat on meat and skin on chicken, full-fat dairy foods, deli meats and most commercial cakes, confectionery and biscuits (cookies)
Monounsaturated fat	olives and olive oil, avocados, peanuts and peanut oil, canola oil, macadamia nuts, hazelnuts, pecan nuts, cashew nuts and almonds
Omega-6 polyunsaturated fats	sunflower, safflower, soya bean, sesame, cotton seed and grape seed oils, pine nuts and brazil nuts
Omega-3 polyunsaturated fats	oily types of fish—herring, sardine, mackerel, salmon and tuna; walnuts, canola oil, linseeds and linseed oil, lean red meat and a range of fortified commercial foods
Trans fats	margarines and fat spreads (some countries have less trans fats in these than others), deep-fried fast food, commercial cakes, pastries, pies and biscuits (cookies)

resistance, something you want to avoid if you want good blood glucose control. Therefore, of equal importance to the amount of fat you eat, is the type of fat you eat. So, you need to control both the amount and types of fat you eat.

There are several different types of fats found in food. Some are healthy, some are not. Saturated fat makes insulin resistance worse and blood glucose harder to control. Saturated and trans fats increase your blood cholesterol level, which increases the risk of heart disease. When you have diabetes, your risk of heart problems is already higher than the average person. It is vital you use diet to help and not hinder in this regard.

It is important to make better choices about the types of fats you include in your diet. Small amounts of the healthier poly- and monounsaturated fats won't increase your blood cholesterol or worsen insulin resistance. This means that your blood vessels will stay in better shape and your blood glucose will be easier to control. Omega-3 fats also have unique health benefits when you have diabetes. They help keep your blood more fluid, reduce blood vessel inflammation and keep the heart beating more steadily. Eating oily fish at least three to four times a week will ensure you get enough of these valuable fats in your diet to reap their rewards.

Once you have made the switch to healthier fats, it is important to also consider ways of cutting down on your total fat intake. This is especially important if you are

Tips to reduce saturated fat
- avoid using butter, lard, cream, sour cream, coconut milk or cream and hard cooking margarines
- choose lean meat and trim fat before cooking
- always take the skin off chicken and other poultry
- eat cheese less often and choose lower fat varieties
- avoid high-fat processed deli meats like devon, chicken loaf, salami
- use low- or reduced-fat milk, yoghurt, ice cream and custard
- avoid deep-fried takeaway foods as well as pies, sausage rolls and pasties
- choose tomato-based sauces over creamy types
- eat less commercial biscuits (cookies), cakes, pastries and puddings—save them for special occasions
- use low-fat cooking methods; steaming, grilling, dry frying, baking and barbecuing

watching your weight or need to lose weight. See the tips on the left for the best ways to do this.

Healthy carbohydrates and the glycaemic index

Carbohydrate foods are broken down into glucose after you eat them, providing your body with its main source of energy or fuel. Carbohydrates are the only part of the food you eat that will directly affect your blood glucose level, so the amount and type of carbohydrate you eat plays a big role in your blood glucose control.

Carbohydrates come in three forms: starch, sugar and fibre; which are found in varying proportions in different carbohydrate foods. Starches and sugars are digested to provide energy while fibre (which is largely undigested) keeps the digestive system healthy.

In the past, starches found in foods such as white bread, rice, potato and pasta were called 'complex' carbohydrates because they are large and complex molecules. Sugars like glucose, sucrose, fructose and lactose were called 'simple' carbohydrates because of their small and more simple structure.

Previously, scientists assumed that simple carbohydrates found in food would cause a greater rise in blood glucose than the complex carbohydrates. This was based on the assumption that the smaller sugars would be digested and absorbed faster than the larger starch molecules. This is the reason why people with diabetes were advised to avoid sugar. It was also assumed that the main factor in determining a carbohydrate's effect on blood glucose was the total amount you ate. Subsequently, people with diabetes were given long lists that showed different foods containing the same amount of carbohydrate that could be exchanged for one another in meals and snacks.

In the 1980s when scientists actually measured blood glucose levels in people, they found that the amount of carbohydrate wasn't a good guide to a food's effect on blood glucose. Instead, it was the type of starch or sugar in the food that appeared to have the greatest influence. With this understanding came the realization that the terms 'simple' and 'complex' told us nothing about the way carbohydrates actually behave in the body.

Research into the effect of different carbohydrate foods on blood glucose has continued since these first studies in the 1980s. The Glycaemic Index (GI) emerged from this research—a measure of the extent to which different carbohydrate foods and drinks cause the blood glucose level to rise after they have been eaten. The GI method assigns carbohydrate foods a number from 0 to 100 according to how they cause your blood sugar level to rise after eating them.

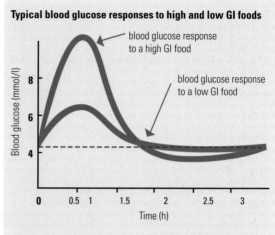

Typical blood glucose responses to high and low GI foods

This graph shows how the body's blood glucose response to high and low-GI foods differs. Quickly-digested, high-GI foods produce a rush of glucose and insulin into the blood-stream followed by a large drop in blood glucose due to the action of insulin. In contrast, a low-GI food results in a smaller rise and fall in blood glucose.

The GI method has shown that some carbohydrate foods like bread, rice and potatoes are digested and absorbed very quickly—far quicker than sugar—and as such have a much greater effect on your blood glucose level than was previously thought. High-GI foods are quickly digested and absorbed and produce a large, rapid rise in blood glucose. Low-GI foods are digested and absorbed more slowly resulting in a less dramatic and more steady blood glucose response and a lower insulin response. The effects of low-GI foods are what is preferred when you have diabetes.

It is difficult to predict the GI of a food just by looking at it, because there are several factors that affect the rate at which carbohydrate is digested:

• **Starch type:** some starches are digested more slowly than others. Foods that contain a greater proportion of slowly digested starch will have a lower GI. For example, basmati rice and the newer specially bred doongara rice have a lower GI

GI ranking categories
Low-GI foods: less than 55
Medium-GI foods: 56 to 69
High-GI foods: greater than 70

than most other rice types because of its higher proportion of slower digested starch.

- **Starch particle size:** the processing of cereals from wholegrain to fine-milled grain makes starch particles smaller and easier to digest and increases their GI. This is why wholegrain breads have a lower GI than wholemeal or finely processed white bread and traditional wholegrain oats have a lower GI than quick-cooking oats.

- **Cooking:** this swells starch particles making them more digestible and raising GI. Overcooked pasta will have a greater GI than when it is cooked *al dente*.

- **Fibre:** soluble fibre found in barley, oats, psyllium, legumes (lentils, chickpeas and dried beans) and some fruits slows digestion by increasing the thickness of food in the stomach.

- **Fat:** slows down food digestion and hence lowers GI. This should not be used as a green light to indulge in unhealthy high-fat foods like chocolate, potato chips (crisps), premium ice creams and croissants. Fatty foods, even if they're low GI, should be limited.

- **Protein:** makes it harder for digestive enzymes to reach starch particles and so slows their digestion. This partly explains why legumes have such a low GI.

- **Acid:** in certain amounts acid can slow food digestion. A salad with vinegar dressing can lower the GI of a meal because of this effect.

A low GI doesn't automatically make a food healthy (as in the case of high-fat foods) and a high-GI food is not always unhealthy. Many high-GI foods such as watermelon, rockmelon and potatoes can still be eaten in moderation if you have diabetes. Simply enjoy them in smaller amounts, less frequently. Eating higher GI foods together with low GI foods will also help lessen their impact on your blood glucose.

Eating low-GI foods as part of a healthy diet and lifestyle, when you have diabetes or pre-diabetes, has many health benefits to offer: lower blood cholesterol and triglycerides; a lower risk of heart problems; blood glucose can be better managed and your body's needs for insulin reduced; and weight loss is easier.

Achieving a lower GI diet is easy using the table of lower and higher GI foods on page 19. Start gradually by making one high-for-low GI food swap each day. Over time, increase the number of foods you swap to one at each meal or snack. You can also try 'diluting' high-GI foods with low-GI foods, for example, have rice with lentils or kidney beans. You can also substitute lower GI ingredients in baking recipes, for example, using stoneground flour instead of refined white flour.

Good GI guide: The foods listed in this table are all healthy carbohydrate foods. However, by eating from the lower GI foods list more often you will find blood glucose control easier and weight more manageable.

HIGH VERSUS LOW GI

Type of food	Higher GI Versions	Lower GI Alternatives
Bread	Regular soft textured white, wholemeal or rye bread and bread rolls, white or wholemeal bagels, gluten-free bread, lebanese bread, melba toast, scones	Wholegrain breads with a relatively dense texture, pumpernickel bread, pitta bread, sourdough bread, breads made from coarse stoneground flour
Grains	Most types of rice (especially jasmine), millet, polenta (cornmeal)	Basmati rice, doongara rice, pearled barley, quinoa, buckwheat, bulgur (cracked wheat)
Pasta and noodles	Gluten-free corn or rice pasta, low-fat instant noodles, dried rice noodles, udon noodles, couscous	Durum wheat pasta—regular or protein-enriched, gluten-free legume-based pasta, mung bean noodles, fresh rice noodles, soba noodles, tortellini, ravioli
Breakfast cereals	Most processed breakfast cereals, including puffed grains (rice, amaranth, wheat, buckwheat), instant porridge, regular wheat breakfast biscuit cereals	Semolina, porridge made from whole or steel-cut oats, oat bran, natural muesli (without flakes), oat bran wheat biscuits
Biscuits and crackers *	Puffed crispbreads, water biscuits, wafer biscuits, plain sweet biscuits: morning coffee biscuits	Biscuits (cookies) made with stoneground flour, whole rolled oats or whole grains with low-GI dried fruit
Vegetables and legumes **	Pumpkin, parsnips, swede, tapioca; most potatoes—steamed, boiled, mashed (new potatoes have the lowest GI value out of the common varieties tested so far, but are still medium GI)	Sweet potato, yams, taro, green peas, carrots, sweet corn, all legumes (dried, boiled, canned, vacuum-packed); non-starchy vegetables (e.g. onions, tomatoes, lettuce, mushrooms, artichokes, asparagus, broccoli, cauliflower, ginger, garlic, cucumber, celery, capsicum (pepper), leeks, herbs
Fruit	Rockmelon, watermelon, sweetened dried cranberries, raisins, dried tenderized figs, lychees, canned in syrup, dark cherries, breadfruit, paw paw	Apples, pears, stone fruit (raw or canned in natural juice), berries, bananas (the less ripe, the lower the GI), prunes, dried apples, apricots, peaches, pears, sultanas, kiwi fruit, mango, custard apple, citrus fruit, grapes
Dairy products and alternatives ***	Rice milk, sweetened condensed milk	Cows milk—plain or flavoured, all types, soy milk—plain or flavoured, all types, yoghurt, ice cream, custard pudding, fromage frais, diet jelly

  * Some biscuits and crackers have low-GI values due to their high fat content, and should not be eaten regularly.
 ** Most vegetables and herbs contain a little carbohydrate and don't produce a marked rise in blood glucose.
*** Dairy products that are sweetened with sugar have a higher GI value than those sweetened with a low-calorie sugar substitute.

More on sweeteners
Sweeteners are not all the same. Some are calorie free and won't affect your blood glucose level (non-nutritive or intense sweeteners), while others have a similar amount of calories to regular table sugar but have varying effects on your blood glucose (nutritive or carbohydrate-modified sweeteners). Similarly, some sweeteners can be used in your cooking (aspartame and sucralose) while others can't. Concerns are raised from time to time about the safety of intense sweeteners. All sweeteners used in foods and drinks have been thoroughly tested before being approved by government food regulators and can be considered safe when using in normal amounts. It is recommended during pregnancy and breastfeeding however, that you use only aspartame and sucralose or foods sweetened with them.

Eat regular meals based on wholegrain and low-GI carbohydrate foods

Your diabetes will be easier to manage if you eat regular meals each day. For some this may mean three modest sized meals—breakfast, lunch and dinner—while for others it may mean four to five smaller meals and snacks. Either way, it's best to avoid large amounts of carbohydrate-containing food at any one time of the day becaues this will make it harder for your body to keep your blood glucose level in the normal range.

Basing your meals on wholegrain, low-GI carbohydrate foods, lean protein, fruit, vegetables and healthy fats will help keep your blood glucose level in the normal range—and help keep hunger at bay.

For anyone with diabetes, especially if you need tablets or insulin, the advice of a dietitian is essential. A dietitian can help you work out the type of eating plan best suited to your health, medication and lifestyle needs.

Include lean protein foods

Protein foods are important for the maintenance and repair of body cells. These foods are also good sources of the minerals iron and zinc, and vitamins B12 and niacin. The best protein foods are lean meat, poultry, fish, eggs, nuts, legumes and seeds.

With all the hype over high-protein, low-carbohydrate diets and the belief that they promote weight loss, it is important to understand how these diets may harm your diabetes before you consider starting one. High-protein, low-carbohydrate diets should always be used with care when you have diabetes. This is especially so when you need insulin or tablets to manage your blood glucose.

Problems with high-protein, low-carbohydrate diets include:

• An increased risk of hypoglycaemia (low blood glucose)

- An increased saturated fat intake which puts you at greater risk of high blood cholesterol levels and heart problems
- More protein in your diet may harm your kidneys, especially if they are already damaged.

However, if you are in good health and are finding your weight hard to shift, more lean protein and a little less carbohydrate on your plate may help. Especially if the carbohydrate you eat is low GI. This isn't, however, a high-protein, low-carbohydrate diet. Consult with a dietitian for more advice if you are having trouble controlling your weight.

Watch the sugar and sugary foods

Too much sugar does not cause diabetes. People with diabetes no longer need to go to extreme lengths to avoid sugar like they used to. This is because research has shown us that sugar has a medium GI and has only a moderate effect on blood glucose (lower than some starchy foods like white or wholemeal bread). Today, sugar is considered a part of a healthy diet for diabetes. However, it is still important to take care with added sugars as they are a source of extra calories.

Low carbohydrate vegetables
Asian greens e.g. bok choy (pak choy), Chinese broccoli (gai larn), choy sum
Asparagus
Broccoli
Brussels sprouts
Cabbage
Capsicum (pepper)
Cauliflower
Celery
Cucumber
Eggplant (aubergine)
Garlic
Leeks
Lettuce
Onions
Mushrooms
Radish
Rocket (arugula)
Spinach
Squash (baby (pattypan) squash)
Watercress
Zucchini (courgettes)

A little brown sugar added to porridge, jam on grainy bread, or added sugar in low-fat yoghurt are healthy ways to include sugar everyday and are unlikely to have a dramatic effect on your blood glucose level. (However, it is sensible to use 'diet' varieties of foods like yoghurt and jam sweetened with low-calorie sweeteners if you're trying to lose weight and are having difficulty keeping your blood glucose under control.) On the other hand, too much added sugar from non-diet soft drinks, fruit juice, lollies, chocolates, cakes and biscuits (cookies) probably will. These higher sugar foods are also more likely to contribute excess calories, and make managing your weight much more difficult.

While it is not always necessary to use an alternative to sugar, there is still a place for sweeteners and sweetened foods in your diet when you have diabetes. However,

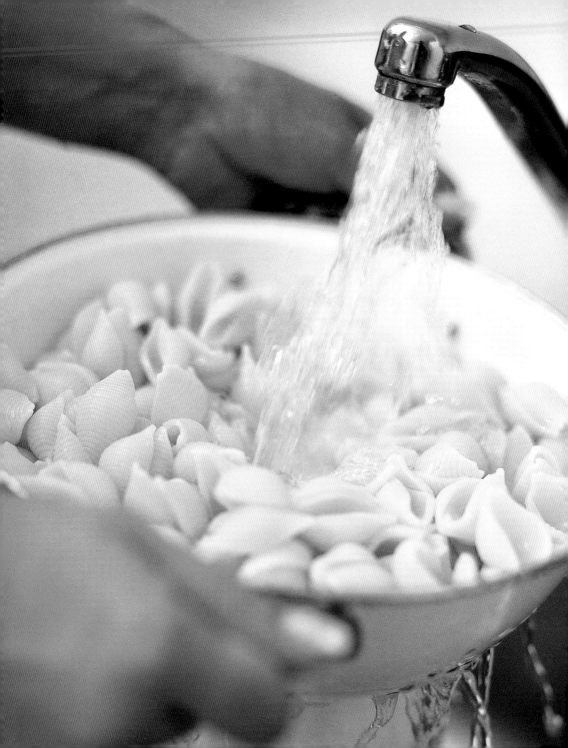

using diet products and low-calorie sweeteners more often than sugar-sweetened versions is still a good idea. Baking is also a good opportunity to use sweeteners, such as sucralose, and there are several products available that replace sugar spoon for spoon to give equal sweetness but with less calories.

Eat more vegetables and legumes

Everyone needs at least five serves of vegetables every day. Unfortunately, most of us don't eat enough, and if you have diabetes you are probably no exception! Increasing your vegetable intake has several benefits:

- It will help you feel full with fewer calories—if you need to cut back on your food intake and have a big appetite, try a leafy salad with a low fat dressing as an entrée.
- You will eat more fibre, which helps improve regularity and blood glucose and cholesterol levels
- It will help protect your eyes and blood vessels from the damage caused by high blood glucose levels—the antioxidants and other protective phytochemicals in vegetables, herbs, spices and fruits have been shown to help protect our eyes.

Don't hold back, load up your plate at every opportunity. Low-carbohydrate types are best, especially if you need to manage your weight, and, the brighter the colour the better for important protective antioxidants and phytochemicals.

Shop smart

Being a smart shopper and choosing the healthiest foods for you requires some skill in reading food labels. When comparing products always use the per 100 g (3½ oz) column of the nutrition information panel found on the pack.

Fat: Choose foods that are lowest in fat and don't forget to check out their saturated fat levels. Occasionally it is OK to choose higher fat foods if their saturated fat is very low and they mostly contain poly- or monounsaturated fats.

Sugar: The total amount of sugar in a food includes added sugars and those occurring naturally such as that from fruit or milk. Go for lower sugar foods where you can.

Fibre: Always choose foods with the most fibre. High fibre foods have 3 g of fibre per serve while very high fibre foods have 6 g or more fibre per serve.

Salt: Look for salt-reduced or no-added-salt foods wherever you can. As a guide foods with less than 120 mgs of sodium per 100 g are good choices.

GI: Choose foods with oats, wholegrains, nuts, seeds, rice bran or oat bran, dried fruit. Also, keep an eye out for the GI symbol on foods, but consider their fat and calorie content before you buy. Not all processed low-GI foods are helpful for weight control.

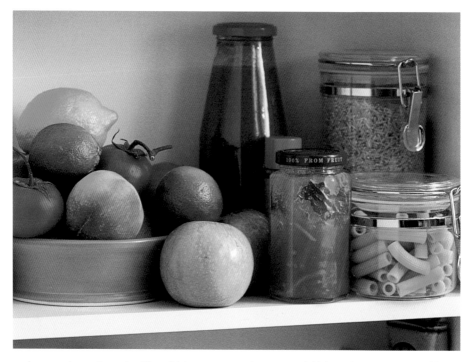

Legumes such as lentils, chickpeas, soya beans and kidney beans are nutritious, low-GI and high in fibre and antioxidants and should be a staple in your pantry—and can easliy be added to soups, casseroles and salads.

Keep salt down

Too much salt can raise your blood pressure, increasing your risk of heart and kidney problems. Simply avoiding adding salt while cooking or to your meals is not enough. Around 75 per cent of the salt in our diets comes from processed foods.

To keep salt down, look for reduced-salt or no-added-salt versions of the foods you normally buy. You will most commonly find lower salt alternatives for margarine spreads, canned tomatoes, tomato paste, tomato sauce, baked beans, cracker biscuits, peanut butter, cheese and cooking stocks or sauces. Always drain and rinse tinned legumes and buy fish in water, not brine or oil.

Avoiding obviously salty foods, such as bacon, ham, olives, canned fish in brine, salted nuts and chips (crisps) will also help keep your salt intake down.

Enjoy alcohol in moderation

Alcohol guidelines for people with diabetes are similar to those for people without diabetes: two to three standard drinks a day with a few alcohol-free days each week. However, if you have diabetes, it is always better to enjoy alcohol with a meal or some carbohydrate food.

Alcohol is high in calories making it harder to manage your weight. It also increases triglycerides (a type of blood fat) and blood pressure, and can cause your blood glucose to go dangerously low (a hypo) if you use insulin or tablets to control your diabetes. Therefore, it is better for your health and blood glucose control if you watch your alcohol intake and reduce it where you can.

Before considering the place of alcohol in your life, discuss its pros and cons with your doctor, diabetes educator or dietitian. This is especially important if you use tablets or insulin to manage your diabetes, as alcohol may not be safe unless you are combining it with the right amounts of carbohydrate.

Simple tips to cut back on alcohol include:

- Reducing your thirst before you drink alcohol with water or diet drinks
- Drink low-alcohol beer
- Alternate alcoholic and non-alcoholic drinks
- Dilute alcoholic drinks such as wine with soda or a beer with diet lemonade

Exercise, a final word ...

A cookbook is obviously about what you eat. However, no advice about health, diet and weight is complete without some mention of physical activity. If you have or are at risk of diabetes then becoming more physically active is vital to achieving the lifestyle you need to optimize your health.

Advantages to being more physically active include:

- Better insulin sensitivity so your body needs less insulin
- Lowers blood pressure
- Helps lower blood cholesterol
- Makes weight control easier
- Reduces stress
- Strengthens your bones and muscles
- Makes you feel good

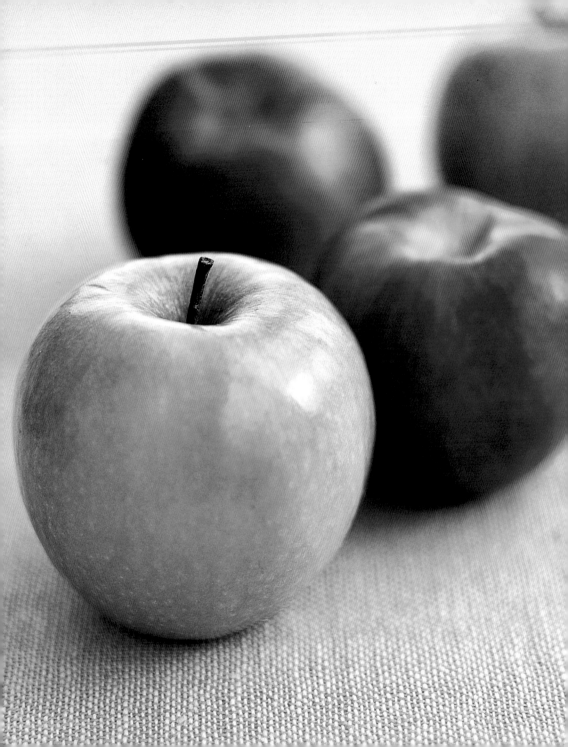

For advice on the amount and type of physical activity you need it is best to consult with your doctor, exercise physiologist or diabetes educator. These health professionals are most able to consider what exercise is appropriate for you given your medical background and current level of fitness.

Being aware of how active you are in your normal daily routine can also help you make changes to how you do things. Investing in a pedometer will tell you about the number of steps you take each day. The more steps you take, the more physically active you become. Think of ways to increase your daily physical activity, such as:

- Taking the stairs rather than the lift or escalator
- Parking a little further away from the doors at the shopping mall
- Walking to get the paper rather than taking the car
- Getting up to turn the TV off rather than using the remote
- Making a regular date with a friend to go for a walk.

How to use this book

The recipes in this book have all been selected because of the valuable contribution they make to healthy eating. Any higher fat recipes are rich in heart friendly monounsaturated or polyunsaturated fats. Where possible the recipes are also high in fibre and contain low glycaemic index (GI) carbohydrates to make blood glucose levels easier to manage. All of the recipes are low in saturated fat to help reduce your risk of heart desease.

Disclaimer

The information in this book is intended to provide people with diabetes, and people who care for them, with general advice about healthy low-GI eating (accurate at the time of printing). This advice may not be sufficient for some people with multiple health problems or serious complications. It is not intended to replace any advice given to you by a qualified doctor or other mainstream health professional. It is important that diabetes is diagnosed by a doctor, using standard diagnostic tests (blood samples, biopsies and assessment of your symptoms). Neither the author nor the publishers can be held responsible for claims arising from the inappropriate use or incorrect interpretation of any of the dietary advice described in this book.

BREAKFAST

HOME-MADE MUESLI

NATURAL MUESLI PROVIDES A HEALTHY MIX OF NUTRIENTS AND DELICIOUS FLAVOURS. SERVED WITH FRESH FRUIT, MILK OR YOGHURT IT'S A GREAT WAY TO START THE DAY.

200 g (7 oz/2 cups) wholegrain rolled (porridge) oats

2 tbsp wheat germ

20 g (¾ oz/¼ cup) unprocessed wheat bran or oat bran

90 g (3¼ oz/½ cup) dried apricots, chopped

35 g (1¼ oz/½ cup) dried apple, chopped

40 g (1½ oz/⅓ cup) sultanas (golden raisins)

60 g (2¼ oz/½ cup) slivered raw almonds

low-fat milk, to serve

PREP TIME: 10 MINUTES

COOKING TIME: NIL

SERVES 8

Combine the rolled oats, wheat germ, wheat bran, dried fruit and almonds in a bowl and mix well. Store in an airtight container until ready to use.

Serve the muesli with low-fat milk.

HINTS:
- This muesli can be stored in an airtight container for up to 4 weeks.
- It will be low GI as long as you use wholegrain oats not quick-cooking oats (the white ones you get in supermarkets). You can substitute the almonds with Brazil nuts, hazelnuts or pecans.
- To save preparation time, you can buy a packet of chopped dried fruit medley to use instead of the apricot, apple and sultanas. Replace the sultanas with lower GI dried pear, peach or prunes, if you prefer.
- For some low-GI serving suggestions, try low-fat yoghurt or fresh low-GI fruit, such as berries, apple, pear, peach, plum, apricot or nectarine.

nutrition per serve: Energy 840 kJ (201 Cal); Fat 6.2 g; Saturated fat 0.7 g; Protein 5.5 g; Carbohydrate 28.2 g; Fibre 5.4 g; Cholesterol 0 mg

BIRCHER MUESLI

IF YOUR REGULAR MUESLI IS A BIT HO-HUM, TRY THIS ONE. IT'S NOT ONLY DELICIOUS, IT'S LOW GI, FILLING AND A GOOD SOURCE OF SOLUBLE FIBRE AND PRODUCES A RANGE OF VITAMINS AND MINERALS.

300 g (10½ oz/3 cups) wholegrain rolled (porridge) oats

250 ml (9 fl oz/1 cup) low-fat milk

100 g (3½ oz/⅓ cup) low-fat plain yoghurt

100 ml (3½ fl oz) freshly squeezed unsweetened orange juice

about 2 cups mixed seasonal fresh low-GI fruit, such as ripe banana, peach, pear, plum, apple or berries

2 apples, grated

125 g (4½ oz/½ cup) low-fat plain yoghurt, extra

1 tbsp pure maple syrup, to serve (optional)

PREP TIME: 15 MINUTES +
4 HOURS REFRIGERATION
COOKING TIME: NIL
SERVES 6

Combine the oats, milk, yoghurt and orange juice in a bowl and mix well. Cover and refrigerate for 4 hours, or overnight.

Serve with the low-GI fresh fruit of your choice, grated apple and extra yoghurt. Drizzle with a little maple syrup, if desired.

HINTS:
• Make sure you use wholegrain oats, not quick-cooking ones.
• You can also add 60 g (2¼ oz/½ cup) slivered almonds. This will increase the fat and energy content, but the fat will be mostly the unsaturated type.
• For extra flavour you can add the grated apple to the oat mix and then store it in the fridge overnight.

nutrition per serve: Energy 1247 kJ (298 Cal); Fat 4.5 g; Saturated fat 0.8 g; Protein 10 g; Carbohydrate 51.3 g; Fibre 5.6 g; Cholesterol 3 mg

PORRIDGE

**100 g (3½ oz/1 cup) wholegrain rolled
  (porridge) oats**
**125 ml (4 fl oz/½ cup) low-fat milk, plus
  extra to serve**

PREP TIME: 5 MINUTES
COOKING TIME: 10 MINUTES
SERVES 2

Mix the oats with 375 ml (13 fl oz/1½ cups) of cold water in a small heavy-based saucepan. Stir in the milk and bring to the boil. Cook for about 7 minutes, stirring constantly, until thick and creamy. Serve immediately.

Serve the porridge with low-fat milk. It is delicious with a dried fruit compote (see recipe on page 35).

HINTS:
- The coarser the oats, the lower the GI. When choosing oats, avoid instant or quick-cooking oats—these are not low GI. Choose the traditional wholegrain, slow-cooking oats instead. If you can't find wholegrain oats in the supermarket, look for them in your local health food shop. You could also use steel cut oats or Scotch oats.
- For a delicious fruity porridge, stir 2 tablespoons of chopped dried apricots into the mixture for the last 3 minutes of cooking. Some other low-GI serving suggestions to try are stewed apple, grated pear or apple, wheat germ, oat bran (a good source of soluble fibre), dried apricots, dried apples, prunes or low-fat yoghurt.
- If you need to add some sweetener, use some low-GI fruit or a little yellow box honey, pure maple syrup or low-calorie sweetener.

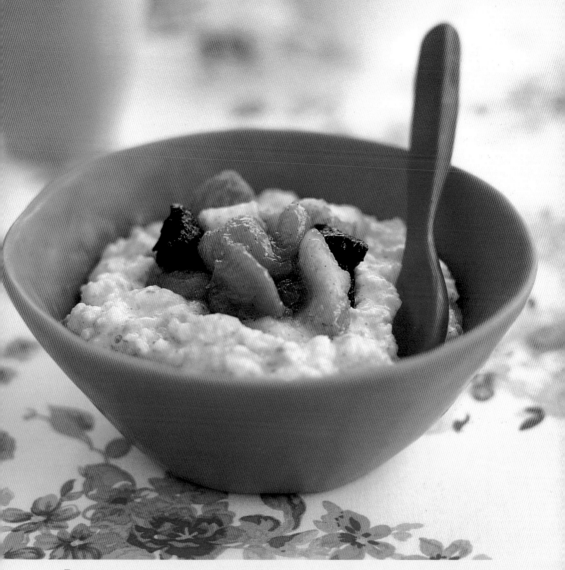

PORRIDGE IS A SUSTAINING BREAKFAST
AND ESPECIALLY NICE TO WARM YOU UP
ON COLD WINTER MORNINGS. USE
TRADITIONAL SLOW-COOKING OATS
INSTEAD OF INSTANT OR QUICK-COOKING
OATS TO KEEP THIS MEAL LOW GI.

nutrition per serve: Energy 915 kJ (219 Cal)
Fat 4.3 g
Saturated fat 0.8 g
Protein 8.1 g
Carbohydrate 34.5 g
Fibre 3.4 g
Cholesterol 3 mg

FRESH FRUIT SALAD

THIS LOW-GI FRESH FRUIT SALAD CAN BE ENJOYED AS A LIGHT MEAL ON ITS OWN—TOPPED WITH SOME LOW-FAT PLAIN YOGHURT AND SUNFLOWER SEEDS OR GROUND LINSEEDS—OR IT CAN BE ADDED TO MUESLI OR EATEN AS SNACK.

2 pears, cored and cut into cubes

2 apples, cored and cut into cubes

120 g (4 oz/¾ cup) strawberries, hulled and halved

120 g (4 oz/¾ cup) blueberries

2 oranges, peeled, seeded and cut into cubes

2 kiwi fruit, peeled and cut into cubes

50 g (1¾ oz/¼ cup) seedless white grapes

2 just-ripe bananas, sliced

3 tbsp unsweetened fruit juice or freshly squeezed orange juice

PREP TIME: 10 MINUTES

COOKING TIME: NIL

SERVES 4

Prepare the fruit just prior to serving. Combine the chopped fruits in a bowl, pour over the fruit juice or orange juice and toss to coat.

HINT:
• You can substitute any seasonal low-GI fruits, such as peaches or mandarins.

nutrition per serve: Energy 911 kJ (218 Cal); Fat 0.4 g; Saturated fat 0 g; Protein 3.4 g; Carbohydrate 46.6 g; Fibre 8.6 g; Cholesterol 0 mg

DRIED FRUIT COMPOTE WITH YOGHURT

THIS FRUITY BREAKFAST IS FULL OF FLAVOUR AND IS A GREAT SOURCE OF FIBRE, CALCIUM AND POTASSIUM. IT ALSO PROVIDES SOME ANTIOXIDANTS, SUCH AS BETACAROTENE. DON'T OVERDO IT THOUGH, IT'S NOT LOW IN CALORIES!

50 g (1¾ oz/⅓ cup) dried apricots, quartered
50 g (1¾ oz/¼ cup) stoned prunes, quartered
50 g (1¾ oz/⅓ cup) dried pears, chopped
50 g (1¾ oz/⅓ cup) dried peaches, chopped
185 ml (6 fl oz/¾ cup) freshly squeezed orange juice

1 cinnamon stick
low-fat plain yoghurt, to serve

PREP TIME: 5 MINUTES
COOKING TIME: 10 MINUTES
SERVES 4

Put the fruit, orange juice and cinnamon stick in a saucepan over medium heat and stir to combine. Bring to the boil, then reduce the heat to low. Cover and simmer for 10 minutes, or until the fruit is plump and softened. Discard the cinnamon stick. Serve drizzled with the cooking liquid and a dollop of the plain yoghurt.

Store in an airtight container in the refrigerator for up to 1 week.

HINT:
• This is a healthy recipe, but people with diabetes should not have large serves because it is an energy-dense food.

nutrition per serve: Energy 525 kJ (125 Cal); Fat 0.2 g; Saturated fat 0 g; Protein 1.9 g; Carbohydrate 27.1 g; Fibre 4.5 g; Cholesterol 0 mg

THIS DISH IS A FANTASTIC
ALTERNATIVE TO BREAKFAST
CEREAL OR PORRIDGE AND IS A
GOOD WAY TO ADD QUINOA
(PRONOUNCED KEEN-WA) TO
YOUR DIET.

nutrition per serve: Energy 1515 kJ (362 Cal)
Fat 3.4 g
Saturated fat 0.3 g
Protein 11.9 g
Carbohydrate 64.6 g
Fibre 9 g
Cholesterol 2 mg

MIXED BERRY QUINOA

200 g (7 oz/1 cup) quinoa, rinsed and
  drained
500 ml (17 fl oz/2 cups) unsweetened
  apple and blackcurrant juice
1 cinnamon stick
250 g (9 oz/2 cups) raspberries
250 g (9 oz/1²⁄₃ cups) blueberries
250 g (9 oz/1²⁄₃ cups) strawberries, hulled
  and halved
2 tsp lime or lemon zest, plus extra

1 tbsp finely shredded mint
200 g (7 oz) low-fat plain or fruit-flavoured
  yoghurt (see Hint)
1 tbsp pure maple syrup (optional)

PREP TIME: 10 MINUTES + REFRIGERATION
  TIME
COOKING TIME: 15 MINUTES
SERVES 4–6

Put the apple and blackcurrent juice and quinoa into a saucepan and add the cinnamon stick. Bring to the boil, then cover and simmer for 12–15 minutes, or until quinoa is translucent and the juice has been absorbed. Remove the cinnamon stick. Transfer to a large bowl, cover and refrigerate until cold.

Add the berries, lime or lemon zest and mint to the quinoa and gently fold through. Spoon the mixture into 4 bowls. Top with a large dollop of yoghurt and a little maple syrup, if desired. Serve chilled.

HINT:
• Flavoured yoghurt with no added sugar has less carbohydrate and calories in it
  and a lower GI than sugar-sweetened yoghurt.

POACHED EGGS WITH SPINACH

THIS EASY RECIPE GIVES YOU A NEW TWIST ON POACHED EGGS WITH MORE FLAVOUR AND NUTRIENTS, AND FAR LESS FAT THAN EGGS BENEDICT. IT'S AN IDEAL MEAL TO ENJOY WITH FRIENDS ON LAZY WEEKENDS.

DRESSING
125 g (4½ oz/½ cup) low-fat plain yoghurt
1 small garlic clove, crushed
1 tbsp chopped chives

300 g (10½ oz) baby English spinach leaves
1 scant tablespoon reduced-fat olive or
   canola oil margarine

4 tomatoes, halved
1 tbsp white vinegar
8 eggs
8 thick slices wholegrain bread, toasted

PREP TIME: 10 MINUTES
COOKING TIME: 15 MINUTES
SERVES 4

To make the dressing, mix together the yoghurt, garlic and chives.

Wash the spinach and put it in a large saucepan with just the little water that is left clinging to the leaves. Cover the pan and cook over low heat for 3–4 minutes, or until the spinach has wilted. Add the margarine, then season with freshly ground black pepper and toss together. Remove the pan from the heat and keep warm.

Put the tomatoes, cut side up, under a preheated grill (broiler) and grill for 3–5 minutes, or until softened and warm.

Fill a deep frying pan three-quarters full with cold water and add the vinegar to stop the egg whites spreading. Bring the water to a gentle simmer. Gently break an egg into a small bowl, then carefully slide into the water, then repeat with the remaining eggs. Reduce the heat so that the water barely moves. Cook for 1–2 minutes, or until the eggs are just set. Remove with a spatula. Drain on paper towels.

Top each slice of toast with some spinach, an egg and some dressing. Serve with the tomato halves. Season with pepper if desired.

nutrition per serve: Energy 1836 kJ (439 Cal); Fat 16.1 g; Saturated fat 4 g; Protein 26.1 g; Carbohydrate 42.3 g; Fibre 8.3 g; Cholesterol 377 mg

MUSHROOMS WITH SCRAMBLED EGGS AND TOMATOES

THIS IS A CLASSIC BREAKFAST, AND FILLING AS WELL! IT PROVIDES GOOD AMOUNTS OF PROTEIN, VITAMIN A, IRON AND FOLATE.

4 field mushrooms

olive or canola spray oil

4 roma (plum) tomatoes, halved

3 tbsp balsamic vinegar

4 eggs, lightly beaten

4 egg whites, lightly beaten

3 tbsp low-fat milk

2 tbsp snipped chives

8 thick slices wholegrain bread

PREP TIME: 10 MINUTES

COOKING TIME: 15 MINUTES

SERVES 4

Trim the mushroom stalks to 2 cm (¾ in) above the cap. Wipe the mushrooms with paper towels to remove any dirt and grit.

Spray both sides of the mushrooms with the oil and place on a non-stick baking tray with the tomatoes. Drizzle the mushrooms and tomatoes with the balsamic vinegar, then sprinkle with freshly ground black pepper and place under a medium grill (broiler) for 10–15 minutes, or until tender.

Meanwhile, put the eggs, egg whites, milk and chives in a bowl and whisk together to combine. Pour the mixture into a non-stick frying pan and cook over a low heat for 2–3 minutes, or until the egg begins to set, then gently stir with a wooden spoon to scramble.

Toast the wholegrain bread until golden brown, then cut on the diagonal. Serve with the mushrooms, tomato and scrambled egg.

HINTS:
- Use omega-3 enriched eggs instead of regular eggs to improve the fat profile of this dish. Omega-3 enriched eggs are available in most large supermarkets and some health food shops.
- People with diabetes are at high risk of developing heart disease (much higher than people without diabetes). So it's important that they don't add salt to their meals.

nutrition per serve: Energy 1399 kJ (334 Cal); Fat 8.5 g; Saturated fat 2 g; Protein 20.8 g; Carbohydrate 39.5 g; Fibre 6.1 g; Cholesterol 188 mg

RICOTTA CORN FRITTERS

200 g (7 oz) low-fat ricotta cheese

1 egg

1 egg white

125 ml (4 fl oz/½ cup) skim milk

75 g (2½ oz/½ cup) wholemeal (whole-
wheat) self-raising flour

420 g (15 oz) tinned corn kernels, drained

3 spring onions (scallions), chopped

2 tbsp snipped chives

olive or canola oil spray

100 g (3½ oz) low-fat ricotta cheese, extra

100 g (3½ oz/⅓ cup) spicy tomato chutney

PREP TIME: 10 MINUTES

COOKING TIME: 25 MINUTES

SERVES 4

Combine the ricotta, egg, egg white and milk in a bowl and beat until smooth. Stir in the flour, corn kernels, spring onion and chives. Season well with freshly ground black pepper.

Spray a non-stick frying pan with the oil. Add heaped tablespoons of the mixture to the pan, four at a time, and flatten to about 1.5 cm (⅝ in) thick. Cook for 3–4 minutes each side. Drain on paper towels.

Serve the fritters in a stack of three and top with a tablespoon of ricotta cheese and a tablespoon of spicy tomato chutney.

HINTS:
• Use stoneground wholemeal flour to help reduce the GI of this dish.
• You could also serve with some grilled tomatoes, mushrooms, spinach and wholegrain bread for a more filling meal.

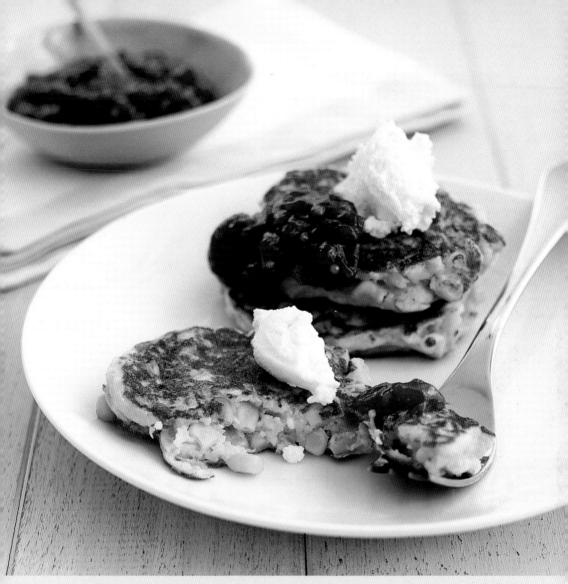

A NICE CHOICE FOR A SAVOURY
BREAKFAST—THIS DELICIOUS,
REDUCED-FAT FRITTER RECIPE
IS A GREAT SOURCE OF
PROTEIN, CALCIUM, VITAMIN A
AND B VITAMINS.

nutrition per serve: Energy 1243 kJ (297 Cal)
Fat 7.2 g
Saturated fat 2.2 g
Protein 15.6 g
Carbohydrate 39.7 g
Fibre 5.4 g
Cholesterol 48 mg

HERB OMELETTE

THIS NOURISHING OMELETTE IS READY IN A FLASH AND IS DELICIOUS AT ANY TIME OF THE DAY. THE COMBINATION OF PROTEIN AND LOW-GI CARBOHYDRATE MAKES IT VERY SUSTAINING.

4 eggs
2 tbsp finely chopped flat-leaf (Italian) parsley
2 tbsp chopped chives
olive or canola oil spray
40 g (1½ oz/⅓ cup) low-fat grated cheddar cheese

4 thick slices wholegrain bread, toasted
fresh cherry tomatoes, to serve

PREP TIME: 10 MINUTES
COOKING TIME: 5 MINUTES
SERVES 2

Break the eggs into a large bowl and whisk with a fork. Whisk in 2 tablespoons of water, then add the parsley and chives. Season with freshly ground black pepper.

Spray a small non-stick frying pan with the oil. Heat over high heat, then reduce the heat to medium and add half of the omelette mixture. Swirl with a fork several times.

While the mixture is cooking, tilt the pan and lift the edge of the omelette occasionally to allow the uncooked egg to flow underneath. When the mixture is half cooked, sprinkle with half of the grated cheese, then leave to cook a little more (the base should be golden brown and the inside nearly set). Using a spatula, fold the omelette in half in the pan. Flip it over onto a warm plate.

Gently re-whisk the remaining egg mixture, then cook in the same way as the first. Serve with the toast and fresh cherry tomatoes.

nutrition per serve: Energy 1708 kJ (408 Cal); Fat 15.6 g; Saturated fat 4.6 g; Protein 27.7 g; Carbohydrate 37 g; Fibre 4.5 g; Cholesterol 382 mg

HOME-MADE BAKED BEANS

Healthier than tinned baked beans, this dish is a delicious way to include more legumes in your diet. Beans are rich in fibre and potassium and the tomatoes are a good source of antioxidants.

550 g (1 lb 4 oz/3 cups) dried haricot beans
400 g (14 oz/1²/₃ cups) no-added salt
   tinned diced tomatoes
250 ml (9 fl oz/1 cup) reduced-salt
   vegetable or chicken stock
1 bay leaf
2 tbsp chopped flat-leaf (Italian) parsley

pinch of dried thyme
1 tbsp olive or canola oil

PREP TIME: 5 MINUTES + 8 HOURS SOAKING
COOKING TIME: 2 HOURS 10 MINUTES
SERVES 4

Wash the beans and place in a large bowl. Cover with 1.5 litres (52 fl oz/6 cups) water and soak for 8 hours, or overnight. Drain.

Cook the haricot beans in a saucepan filled with plenty of water for about 1½ hours, or until tender. Drain. Preheat the oven to 180°C (350°F/Gas 4).

Put the beans in a casserole dish and add the tomato, stock, herbs and oil. Bake, covered, for 40 minutes.

Serve the baked beans with grainy toast or grainy muffins spread with a little low-fat cottage cheese topped with fresh spinach, and season with pepper.

HINTS:
• If you want a thicker consistency, remove the lid of the casserole dish and cook for a further 10–15 minutes, or until reduced to the desired consistency. Instead of using dried haricot beans, you can use the same amount of drained tinned haricot beans.

nutrition per serve: Energy 193 kJ (462 Cal); Fat 8 g; Saturated fat 1.1 g; Protein 31.2 g; Carbohydrate 57.9 g; Fibre 27.7 g; Cholesterol 1 mg

THIS NOURISHING MEAL IS A
GOOD SOURCE OF MANY
NUTRIENTS INCLUDING
PROTEIN, B-GROUP VITAMINS
AND ANTIOXIDANTS. SERVE
WITH WHOLEGRAIN BREAD FOR
A BALANCED LOW-GI MEAL.

nutrition per serve: 1497 kJ (358 Cal)
Fat 15.6 g
Saturated fat 3.9 g
Protein 15 g
Carbohydrate 36.5 g
Fibre 5.4 g
Cholesterol 187 mg

EGGS EN COCOTTE

TOMATO SAUCE
1 tbsp olive or canola oil
1 garlic clove, crushed
3 vine-ripened tomatoes (about 300 g/
 10½ oz), peeled, seeded and chopped

½ tsp olive or canola oil
4 eggs
Tabasco sauce, to taste

2 tbsp snipped fresh chives
8 slices thick wholegrain bread
1 tbsp reduced-fat olive or canola oil
 margarine

PREP TIME: 15 MINUTES
COOKING TIME: 30 MINUTES
SERVES 4

Preheat the oven to 180°C (350°F/Gas 4). To make the tomato sauce, heat the oil in a heavy-based frying pan. Add the garlic and cook for 1 minute, or until it begins to turn golden. Add the tomato and season with some freshly ground black pepper. Cook over medium heat for 15 minutes, or until thickened.

Grease four 125 ml (4 fl oz/½ cup) ramekins with the oil, then break 1 egg into each, trying not to break the yolk. Pour the sauce around the outside of each egg so the yolk is still visible. Add a little tabasco sauce, sprinkle with the chives and season with pepper, if desired.

Place the ramekins in a deep baking dish and pour in enough hot water to come halfway up the side of the ramekins. Bake for 7–10 minutes, or until the egg white is set. Toast the bread and lightly spread with the margarine. Serve immediately with the egg.

SCRAMBLED TOFU WITH MUSHROOMS

THIS IS A NOURISHING LOW-GI BREAKFAST WHICH PROVIDES GOOD AMOUNTS OF PROTEIN, FIBRE, FOLATE AND IRON.

1 tbsp reduced-fat olive or canola oil margarine
200 g (7 oz) button mushrooms, sliced
1 garlic clove, crushed
2 spring onions (scallions), chopped
400 g (14 oz) firm tofu, drained and crumbled

1 tsp reduced-sodium soy sauce
1 tbsp finely chopped flat-leaf (Italian) parsley
8 thick slices soy and linseed bread

PREP TIME: 10 MINUTES
COOKING TIME: 15 MINUTES
SERVES 4

Melt half of the margarine in a large frying pan. Add the mushrooms and cook over high heat for 5 minutes, or until they start to lose their moisture. Add the garlic and cook for 5 minutes, or until the liquid has evaporated. Remove from the pan.

Melt the remaining margarine in the pan. Add the spring onion and cook for 30 seconds, or until just wilted. Add the tofu, soy sauce and mushrooms and cook, stirring gently, for 2 minutes, or until the tofu is heated through. Stir in the parsley and season with freshly ground black pepper.

Lightly toast the bread and serve with the scrambled tofu.

HINT:
• Add some tomatoes and spinach if you want some more flavour and colour.

nutrition per serve: Energy 1525 kJ (364 Cal); Fat 16.7 g; Saturated fat 2.6 g; Protein 26.4 g; Carbohydrate 26.4 g; Fibre 7.8; Cholesterol 0 mg

SUMMER ORANGE JUICE

THIS REFRESHING BLEND OF CITRUS AND STONE-FRUIT JUICES IS A RICH SOURCE OF FOLATE, POTASSIUM AND THE ANTIOXIDANTS BETACAROTENE AND VITAMIN C.

3 oranges, peeled
5 small plums, stones removed
4 peaches, stones removed
10 apricots, stones removed

PREP TIME: 10 MINUTES
COOKING TIME: NIL
SERVES 2

Juice the oranges, plums, peaches and apricots in a juice extractor or blender. Stir well to combine.

HINT:
• Enjoy this juice in moderation if you are watching your weight. Fresh fruit is more filling than fruit juice. The general recommendation for adults and kids is to drink no more than one juice drink a day.

nutrition per serve: Energy 1506 kJ (360 Cal); Fat 1.2 g; Saturated fat 0 g; Protein 7.5 g; Carbohydrate 67.4 g; Fibre 15 g; Cholesterol 0 mg

BANANA SMOOTHIE

2 just-ripe bananas
60 g (2¼ oz/¼ cup) low-fat vanilla or
  fruit-flavoured yoghurt
500 ml (17 fl oz/2 cups) low-fat milk
2 tbsp wheat germ or oat bran
freshly grated nutmeg, to taste

PREP TIME: 5 MINUTES
COOKING TIME: NIL
SERVES 2

Put the bananas in a blender or food processor. Add the yoghurt, milk, wheat germ and nutmeg. Blend or process until smooth, then pour into two chilled glasses.

HINTS:
- The GI of bananas increases as the fruit ripens, so choose bananas that have only just ripened.
- You can substitute the bananas with other low-GI fruit, such as berries, pears, apricots, plums, peaches or nectarines.
- Choose a flavoured yoghurt with no added sugar. Check the ingredients list and look for one that has been sweetened with a low-calorie sweetener, such as aspartame, rather than sugar.
- Choose calcium-enriched, low-fat milk for a calcium boost.

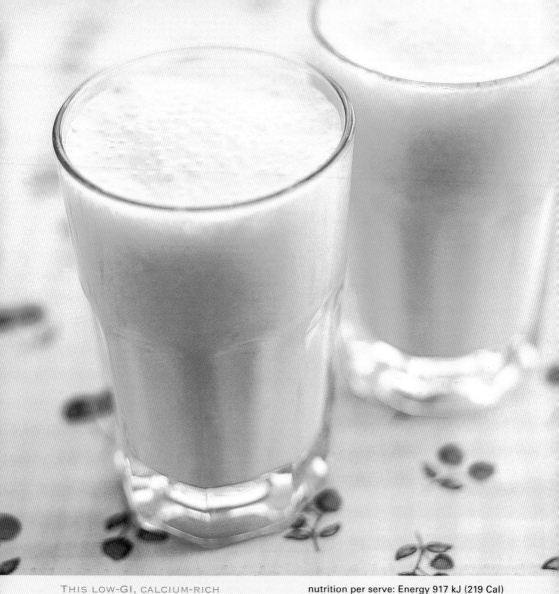

THIS LOW-GI, CALCIUM-RICH
SMOOTHIE IS GOOD FOR YOUR
TEETH AND BONES AND MAKES
A DELICIOUS LIGHT BREAKFAST.

nutrition per serve: Energy 917 kJ (219 Cal)

Fat 1 g

Saturated fat 0.5 g

Protein 14.3 g

Carbohydrate 37.1 g

Fibre 3.4 g

Cholesterol 10 mg

BREAKFAST SMOOTHIE

This refreshing smoothie provides some carbohydrate and protein to help energize your brain and body and improve your mood. It's very easy to make and even easier to drink.

**150 g (5½ oz) fresh low-GI fruit, such as
peach, plum, pear, or strawberries**
60 g (2¼ oz/¼ cup) low-fat vanilla yoghurt
250 ml (9 fl oz/1 cup) low-fat milk
1 tbsp malted milk powder
2 tsp wheat germ or oat bran
1 egg (optional)

PREP TIME: 5 MINUTES
COOKING TIME: NIL
SERVES 2

Put the fruit in a blender or food processor. Add the yoghurt, milk, milk powder, wheat germ and egg (if you are using it). Blend or process until well combined, then pour into two chilled glasses.

HINTS:
- Experiment with various low-GI fruits to work out your favourite combination for this low-fat smoothie.
- There are many types of yoghurt on the market. Choose a low-fat diet yoghurt that contains a low-calorie sweetener instead of sugar. Diet yoghurt that is sweetened with aspartame or a similar low-calorie sweetener has a lower GI and less calories than yoghurt sweetened with sugar.

nutrition per serve: Energy 599 kJ (143 Cal); Fat 3.3 g; Saturated fat 1.1 g; Protein 11.4 g; Carbohydrate 16.3 g; Fibre 1.4 g; Cholesterol 101 mg

CARROT, APRICOT AND NECTARINE JUICE

One vegetable and two fruits combine to make this delicious and nutritious drink, rich in antioxidants.

1 kg (2 lb 4 oz) baby carrots
10 apricots, stones removed
4 large nectarines, stones removed
ice cubes, to serve
lemon slices, to serve

PREP TIME: 10 MINUTES
COOKING TIME: NIL
SERVES 2

Juice the carrots, apricots and nectarines in a juice extractor or use a blender. Stir to combine and serve over ice with lemon slices.

nutrition per serve: Energy 1884 kJ (450 Cal); Fat 1.5 g; Saturated fat 0 g; Protein 10.9 g; Carbohydrate 81 g; Fibre 25; Cholesterol 0 mg

SNACKS AND LIGHT MEALS

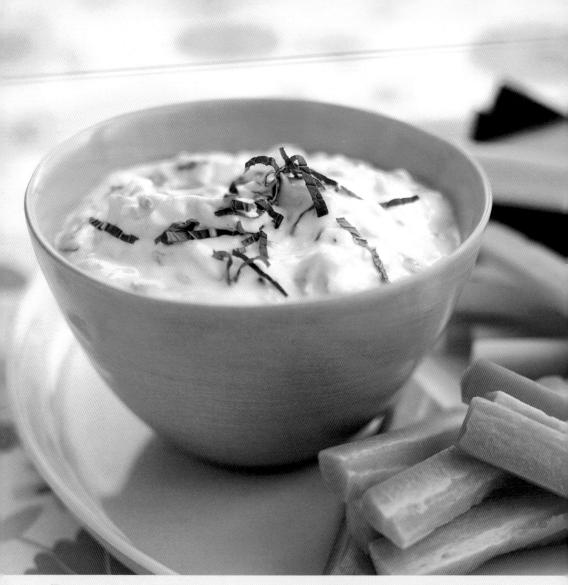

THIS LOW-CALORIE DIP IS
DELICIOUS AS A SNACK WITH
CRUNCHY RAW VEGETABLE
STICKS OR AS A LOW-FAT
SUBSTITUTE FOR MAYONNAISE
OR MARGARINE IN SANDWICHES
AND BURGERS.

nutrition per serve: Energy 93 kJ (22 Cal)
Fat 0.1 g
Saturated fat 0.04 g
Protein 2.2 g
Carbohydrate 2.5 g
Fibre 0.4 g
Cholesterol 2 mg

TZATZIKI

2 Lebanese (short) cucumbers
400 g (14 oz/1²/₃ cups) low-fat
  plain yoghurt
4 garlic cloves, crushed
3 tbsp finely chopped mint, plus extra,
  to garnish
1 tbsp lemon juice

PREP TIME: 10 MINUTES +
  15 MINUTES STANDING
COOKING TIME: NIL
SERVES 12

Cut the cucumbers in half lengthways, scoop out the seeds and discard. Leave the skin on and coarsely grate the cucumber into a small colander. Sprinkle with salt and leave over a large bowl for 15 minutes to drain off any bitter juices.

Meanwhile, combine the yoghurt, garlic, mint and lemon juice.

Rinse the cucumber under cold water then, taking small handfuls, squeeze out any excess moisture. Combine the grated cucumber with the yoghurt mixture and season well with freshly ground black pepper. Garnish with mint. Serve with vegetable sticks.

HINTS:
• Tzatziki will keep in an airtight container in the fridge for 2–3 days.
• To make vegetable sticks, cut raw carrots, celery, zucchini (courgettes) and unpeeled Lebanese (short) cucumbers into 7 cm (2³/₄ in) sticks, and raw cauliflower and broccoli into small florets.

CANNELLINI BEAN AND CHICKPEA DIP

THIS LOW-GI DIP IS A DELICIOUS AND EASY WAY TO EAT BEANS AND CHICKPEAS. ENJOY AS A SNACK WITH FRESH VEGETABLES OR AS A SPREAD ON BREAD.

425 g (15 oz) tinned cannellini (white) beans, rinsed and drained
425 g (15 oz) tinned chickpeas, rinsed and drained
1½ tsp ground cumin
3 garlic cloves, crushed
2 tbsp chopped flat-leaf (Italian) parsley
3 tbsp lemon juice

1 tsp lemon zest
1 tbsp tahini

PREP TIME: 10 MINUTES
COOKING TIME: NIL
SERVES 3–4

Put all the ingredients in a food processor and process for 30 seconds. With the motor still running, slowly add 3 tablespoons hot water to the processor in a thin stream until the mixture is smooth and 'dippable'. Serve at room temperature with vegetable sticks and pitta crisps.

HINT:
• Tahini is a thick paste made of ground sesame seeds. It is available at large supermarkets and health food shops.

nutrition per serve (4): Energy 735 kJ (175 Cal); Fat 4.9 g; Saturated fat 0.7 g; Protein 10.8 g; Carbohydrate 18.7 g; Fibre 8.8 g; Cholesterol 0 mg

HUMMUS

THIS POPULAR DIP IS A GREAT SOURCE OF FIBRE, FOLATE AND POTASSIUM AS WELL AS BEING DELICIOUS.

220 g (7¾ oz/1 cup) dried chickpeas
3 tbsp olive oil
3–4 tbsp lemon juice
2 garlic cloves, crushed
2 tbsp tahini
1 tbsp ground cumin

PREP TIME: 15 MINUTES + 8 HOURS SOAKING
COOKING TIME: 1 HOUR
SERVES 2–4

Soak the chickpeas in water for 8 hours, or overnight. Drain. Put in a saucepan, cover with cold water, bring to the boil and cook for about 50–60 minutes. Drain, reserving 185–250 ml (6–9 fl oz/¾–1 cup) of the cooking liquid.

Place the chickpeas in a food processor with the oil, lemon juice, garlic, tahini and cumin. Blend well until the mixture begins to look thick and creamy. With the motor running, gradually add the reserved cooking liquid until the mixture reaches the desired consistency. Serve with toasted grainy bread, pitta bread, vegetable sticks or use as a spread on sandwiches.

nutrition per serve: Energy 1667 kJ (398 Cal); Fat 23.4 g; Saturated fat 3 g; Protein 13.1 g; Carbohydrate 25 g; Fibre 11.3 g; Cholesterol 0 mg

RICE PAPER ROLLS WITH PRAWNS

20 large cooked prawns (shrimp), peeled
  and deveined
1 small carrot
1 Lebanese (short) cucumber
125 g (4½ oz/1¾ cups) finely shredded
  red cabbage
 8 spring onions (scallions)
1 handful mint, torn
2 handfuls coriander (cilantro) leaves
20 x 16 cm (8 x 6 in) square rice paper
  wrappers

1 long red chilli, seeded, finely chopped
2 tsp grated palm sugar or
  soft brown sugar
1 tbsp rice vinegar
1 tbsp fish sauce
2 tbsp chopped coriander (cilantro) leaves
  and stems

PREP TIME: 20 MINUTES
COOKING TIME: NIL
MAKES 20 (SERVES 4–6)

DRESSING
125 ml (4 fl oz/½ cup) lime juice
2 tbsp sweet chilli sauce
3 garlic cloves, crushed

Cut the prawns into 1 cm (½ in) slices, on the diagonal. Julienne the carrot into 4 cm
(1½ in) lengths. Cut the cucumber into 1 cm (½ in) lengths. Thinly slice the spring onions
on the diagonal. Put the prawns, cabbage, carrot, cucumber, spring onions, mint and
coriander in a large bowl and toss to combine.

To make the dressing, combine all the dressing ingredients in a small bowl and mix well.
Pour 80 ml (2½ fl oz/⅓ cup) of the dressing over the prawn mixture and toss to combine.
Working with one wrapper at a time, dip into a bowl of hot water for 10 seconds, or until
softened, drain, then lay out on a flat surface.

Place 60 g (2¼ oz/¼ cup) of the mixture on one side of the wrapper, leaving a border at
the sides. Fold in the sides and roll up tightly. Cover with a damp cloth and repeat with the
remaining filling and wrappers to make 20 rolls. Serve with the remaining dressing as a
dipping sauce.

HINT:
• Although delicious, these rice paper rolls should be enjoyed in moderation as the rice
  paper itself is medium GI. They are, however, low in fat.

THESE ROLLS ARE A GREAT
SOURCE OF FOLATE AND THE
ANTIOXIDANTS BETACAROTENE
AND VITAMIN C. THE PRAWNS
PROVIDE IODINE AND
SELENIUM—MINERALS MOST
PEOPLE DON'T EAT ENOUGH OF.

nutrition per serve (4): Energy 1326 kJ (317 Cal)

Fat 1.5 g

Saturated fat 0.3 g

Protein 24.5 g

Carbohydrate 47.9 g

Fibre 3.9 g

Cholesterol 150 mg

STUFFED CAPSICUMS

MEDITERRANEAN-STYLE FLAVOURS ENHANCE THE RICE, HAM AND VEGETABLE FILLING IN THE BAKED CAPSICUMS. THIS COLOURFUL MEAL IS LOW GI AND RICH IN ANTIOXIDANTS AND POTASSIUM.

175 g (6 oz) eggplant (aubergine), peeled and diced

1 onion, finely chopped

2 garlic cloves, chopped

400 g (14 oz) no-added-salt tinned chopped tomatoes

1 tsp sugar

1 tbsp dried thyme

1 tsp dried oregano

375 g (13 oz/2 cups) cooked brown basmati rice

50 g (1¾ oz) chopped low-fat ham (we used 97% fat-free) (optional)

125 g (4½ oz) tinned corn kernels, drained

olive or canola oil spray

4 red capsicums (peppers), halved and seeded

60 g (2¼ oz/½ cup) grated low-fat cheddar cheese

PREP TIME: 25 MINUTES

COOKING TIME: 1 HOUR 5 MINUTES

SERVES 4

Preheat the oven to 180°C (350°F/Gas 4). Place the eggplant, onion, garlic and 125 ml (4 fl oz/½ cup) of water in a large, deep, heavy-based frying pan. Bring to the boil, then lower the heat, cover and simmer for 8 minutes, or until softened. Stir once or twice. Remove the lid and simmer until any remaining liquid has evaporated.

Add the tomatoes, sugar and herbs and season well with pepper. Simmer, uncovered, for 8 minutes. Remove from the heat and stir in the rice, ham and corn.

Spray the capsicum shells on the outside with the oil. Fill the capsicum halves with the mixture. Put the capsicums in a large baking dish, pour 250 ml (9 fl oz/1 cup) of water into the dish, cover with foil and bake for 45 minutes, or until the capsicums have softened. Remove the foil and sprinkle each capsicum half with grated cheese. Bake for a further 5 minutes, or until the cheese has melted. Serve with a mixed green salad dressed with vinegar.

HINT:
• You need 150 g (5½ oz/¾ cup) uncooked brown rice to make 375 g (13 oz/2 cups) cooked brown rice.

nutrition per serve: Energy 1240 kJ (296 Cal); Fat 4.5 g; Saturated fat 1.3 g; Protein 14.6 g; Carbohydrate 45.6 g; Fibre 6.6 g; Cholesterol 11 mg

CORN AND CAPSICUM FRITTERS

JUST LIKE SPANISH OMELETTE, THESE FRITTERS CAN ALSO BE SERVED COLD FOR A PICNIC OR PARTY. TRY SERVING THEM WITH A LOW-FAT DIPPING SAUCE.

1 large red capsicum (pepper)
2–3 cobs fresh corn kernels (about
   300 g/10½ oz) or 300 g (10½ oz/
   1½ cups) tinned corn kernels, drained
olive or canola oil, for frying
2 tbsp chopped flat-leaf (Italian) parsley,
   coriander (cilantro) leaves, chives or dill
3 eggs

PREP TIME: 20 MINUTES
COOKING TIME: 10 MINUTES
SERVES 4

Cut the capsicum into large pieces, discarding the seeds and membrane, then chop into small pieces. Cut the kernels from the fresh corn, using a sharp knife. Heat 2 tablespoons of oil in a frying pan. Add the corn and stir over medium heat for 2 minutes. Add the capsicum and stir for a further 2 minutes. Transfer the vegetables to a bowl. Add the herbs and stir well to combine. Beat the eggs in a small bowl with a little freshly ground black pepper. Stir the egg gradually into the vegetable mixture.

Heat a non-stick frying pan over medium heat. Add enough oil to cover the base. Drop large spoonfuls of the vegetable mixture into the oil, a few at a time. Cook the fritters for 1–2 minutes, or until brown. Turn and cook the other side. Drain on paper towels and keep warm while you cook the remainder.

HINTS:
• These fritters may be served with some wholegrain bread and a green salad for lunch, or as an accompaniment to a main course.
• Take care as these fritters contain no flour, so they cook quickly. You want them to still be a little creamy in the middle when done.

nutrition per serve: Energy 998 kJ (238 Cal); Fat 6.8 g; Saturated fat 1.5 g; Protein 11.3 g; Carbohydrate 29.4 g; Fibre 6.8 g; Cholesterol 141 mg

THESE PIZZAS ARE A MUCH
BETTER CHOICE THAN
COMMERCIAL ONES AND A GOOD
EXAMPLE OF HOW YOU CAN
STILL ENJOY YOUR FAVOURITE
FOODS IN MODERATION IF YOU
HAVE DIABETES.

nutrition per serve: Energy 1806 kJ (431 Cal)

Fat 9.4 g

Saturated fat 4.7 g

Protein 25 g

Carbohydrate 58.8 g

Fibre 8.5 g

Cholesterol 28 mg

PITTA PIZZAS

4 large wholemeal (whole-wheat) pitta
   pocket breads
130 g (4¾ oz/½ cup) 99% fat-free tomato
   salsa
½ red onion, thinly sliced
90 g (3¼ oz) mushrooms, thinly sliced
60 g (2¼ oz) low-fat ham (we used 97%
   fat-free), thinly sliced
90 g (3¼ oz/½ cup) black olives in brine,
   rinsed, drained, pitted and chopped

1 tbsp capers, rinsed, drained and chopped
80 g (2¾ oz/½ cup) low-fat feta cheese
10 g (¼ oz/¼ cup) sprigs rosemary
100 g (3½ oz/1 cup) grated light (reduced-
   fat) mozzarella

PREP TIME: 15 MINUTES
COOKING TIME: 20 MINUTES
SERVES 4

Preheat the oven to 200°C (400°F/Gas 6). Place the pitta breads on a large baking tray or on two smaller trays. Spread each with the salsa. Scatter over the onion, mushrooms, ham, olives and capers.

Crumble over the feta and top with the rosemary sprigs and mozzarella. Bake for 20 minutes. Serve immediately.

VARIATIONS:
• Use no-added-salt tomato pasta sauce or salsa sauce on the base, then choose from the following toppings: low-fat ham, pineapple pieces, sliced capsicum (pepper), onion or olives marinated in brine.
• For a meaty topping, try leftover savoury minced (ground) beef or spaghetti bolognaise and low-fat cheddar cheese.
• For a little spice, try salami, corn kernels, sliced green capsicum, onion, tomato and low-fat feta cheese.
• A tasty vegetarian option is artichoke hearts, tomato and zucchini (courgette) slices, ricotta and low-fat feta cheese.
• An easy seafood version uses tuna in springwater, sliced mushroom and capsicum, and low-fat cheddar cheese.

HINT:
• Look for pitta pockets made from stoneground flour as they are lower GI.

CORN AND BACON CRUSTLESS QUICHES

For an occasional treat, these reduced-fat quiches are delicious— all the flavour but less fat than regular quiches.

4 corn cobs
1 tsp olive or canola oil
4 slices low-fat bacon slices (we used 97% fat-free), cut into thin strips
1 small onion, finely chopped
3 eggs, lightly beaten
2 tbsp chopped chives
2 tbsp chopped flat-leaf (Italian) parsley
60 g (2¼ oz/¾ cup) fresh wholegrain breadcrumbs
4 tbsp skim evaporated milk

PREP TIME: 30 MINUTES
COOKING TIME: 40 MINUTES
MAKES 4

Preheat the oven to 180°C (350°F/Gas 4). Lightly grease four 185 ml (6 fl oz/¾ cup) ramekins. Remove the husks from the corn and, using a coarse grater, grate the corn kernels into a deep bowl. There should be about 1½ cups corn flesh and juice.

Heat the oil in a frying pan and cook the bacon and onion for 3–4 minutes, or until the onion softens. Add to the corn in the bowl. Stir in the eggs, chives, parsley, breadcrumbs and evaporated milk and season well with freshly ground black pepper. Spoon into the ramekins.

Put the ramekins in a large baking dish. Add enough hot water to come halfway up the sides of the ramekins. Lay foil loosely over the top. Bake for 25–30 minutes, or until just set.

nutrition per serve: Energy 1182 kJ (282 Cal); Fat 7.4 g; Saturated fat 1.9 g; Protein 17.2 g; Carbohydrate 35.1 g; Fibre 4.9 g; Cholesterol 149 mg

ITALIAN OMELETTE

IF YOU FIND PLAIN OMELETTES A BIT BORING, THIS ITALIAN-FLAVOURED VERSION IS THE THING FOR YOU. SERVE WITH WHOLEGRAIN BREAD FOR A COMPLETE, MORE FILLING LOW-GI MEAL.

150 g (5½ oz) fusilli
1 tsp olive or canola oil
1 onion, finely chopped
125 g (4½ oz) low-fat ham, sliced
6 eggs
3 tbsp low-fat milk
25 g (1 oz/¼ cup) grated parmesan cheese
2 tbsp chopped flat-leaf (Italian) parsley
1 tbsp chopped basil
olive or canola oil spray

60 g (2¼ oz/½ cup) grated low-fat cheddar cheese
wholegrain bread, to serve

PREP TIME: 20 MINUTES
COOKING TIME: 25 MINUTES
SERVES 4

Cook the pasta in a large saucepan of boiling water for 10 minutes, or until *al dente*. Drain and cool.

Heat the oil in a non-stick frying pan. Add the onion and stir over low heat for 5 minutes, or until tender. Add the ham and stir for 1 minute. Transfer to a plate.

Whisk together the eggs and milk and season well with freshly ground black pepper. Stir in the pasta, parmesan, herbs and onion mixture.

Preheat the grill (broiler). Heat the frying pan and spray with oil. Pour the egg mixture into the pan. Sprinkle with the cheddar. Cook over medium heat until the omelette begins to set around the edges, then put the pan under the grill until the omelette is set and lightly browned on top. Cut into wedges and serve with wholegrain bread.

HINTS:
• You can use any short durum wheat pasta.
• Durum wheat pasta has a low-GI value. However, it should not be overcooked. Overcooking pasta until it is soft and soggy makes its starch more digestible and increases its GI value. Pasta should be served *al dente*.

nutrition per serve: Energy 1463 kJ (350 Cal); Fat 13.7 g; Saturated fat 4.9 g; Protein 27.7 g; Carbohydrate 28 g; Fibre 1.7 g; Cholesterol 308 mg

MUSHROOM AND SPINACH FRITTATA

olive or canola oil spray
1 red onion, thinly sliced
50 g (1¾ oz) low-fat bacon (we used 97% fat-free), thinly sliced
3 garlic cloves, crushed
90 g (3¼ oz) mushrooms, thinly sliced
2 zucchini (courgettes), diced
1 handful baby English spinach leaves
4 eggs
60 ml (2 fl oz/¼ cup) skim or no-fat milk

60 g (2¼ oz/½ cup) grated low-fat cheddar cheese
2 tbsp shredded parmesan cheese
2 tbsp basil, thinly shredded

PREP TIME: 20 MINUTES
COOKING TIME: 25 MINUTES + COOLING TIME
SERVES 4

Spray a large non-stick frying pan with oil. Heat the oil, add the onion, bacon and garlic and stir-fry for 4 minutes, or until soft. Add the mushrooms and zucchini and stir-fry for 3 minutes, or until the mushrooms are cooked and any liquid has evaporated. Stir in the spinach and cook until just wilted. Cool.

Whisk together the eggs and milk in a large bowl. Stir in the cheeses, basil and cooled vegetable mixture.

Take a non-stick frying pan with a diameter of 18–20 cm/7–8 in (across the base) and spray with oil. Pour in the mixture and smooth the surface. Cook over a low heat for 10–13 minutes, or until mostly set. Take care not to burn the base.

Preheat a grill (broiler) to medium. Place the pan under the grill and cook for 3–5 minutes, or until firm and lightly browned on top. Serve warm or cold, cut into slices. Season with pepper and serve with a balsamic-dressed salad.

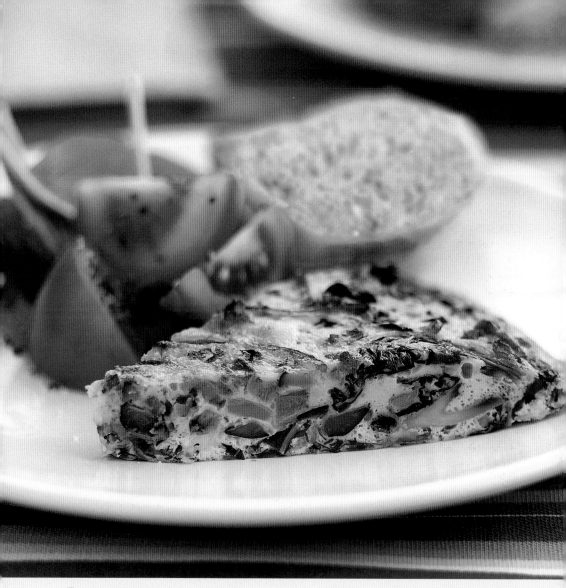

FRITTATAS ARE A FILLING
LIGHT MEAL AND TASTY TO
BOOT! THIS ONE'S A GOOD
SOURCE OF CALCIUM, PROTEIN
AND VITAMINS A, B AND D.

nutrition per serve: Energy 717 kJ (171 Cal)

Fat 9.1 g

Saturated fat 3.3 g

Protein 18 g

Carbohydrate 3.9 g

Fibre 2.3 g

Cholesterol 200 mg

CHICKPEA FRITTERS

THESE LOW-GI FRITTERS ARE AN EXCELLENT SOURCE OF FIBRE AND PROVIDE A GOOD AMOUNT OF PROTEIN TOO.

2 tsp olive or canola oil
4 spring onions (scallions), sliced
2 garlic cloves, finely chopped
1 small red chilli, seeded and finely
    chopped
600 g (1 lb 5 oz) tinned chickpeas, rinsed
    and drained
2 tbsp chopped coriander (cilantro)
1 egg, lightly beaten
olive or canola oil spray

99% fat-free tomato salsa, to serve
100 g (3½ oz) mixed salad leaves, to serve
wholegrain bread, to serve

PREP TIME: 20 MINUTES
COOKING TIME: 25 MINUTES
MAKES 6

Preheat the oven to 200°C (400°F/Gas 6). Line a baking tray with baking paper. Heat 2 teaspoons of the oil in a large non-stick frying pan over medium heat. Add the spring onions, garlic and chilli and cook, stirring, for 1–2 minutes, or until the spring onion softens.

Put the chickpeas and spring onion mixture and coriander in a food processor. Process until the mixture just starts to hold together. Do not overprocess—the mixture should be just roughly processed. Transfer to a bowl and mix in the egg. Using wet hands, shape the mixture into six even fritters.

Lightly spray the fritters with spray oil and put on prepared tray. Bake for 20 minutes turning once until lightly golden brown. Serve with salsa, mixed lettuce and bread.

nutrition per fritter (6): Energy 430 kJ (103 Cal); Fat 4.3 g; Saturated fat 0.7 g; Protein 5.5 g; Carbohydrate 9.1 g; Fibre 3.6 g; Cholesterol 31 mg

BAKED SWEET POTATOES MEXICANA

LIKE SOME SPICE? THIS DISH IS THE PERFECT HOT POTATO! IT CONTAINS CARBOHYDRATE, FIBRE AND ANTIOXIDANTS. TOP WITH LOW-FAT SOUR CREAM OR YOGHURT FOR EXTRA CALCIUM.

4 x 200 g (7 oz) orange sweet potatoes
olive or canola oil spray
1 garlic clove, crushed
1 onion, finely chopped
250 g (9 oz) lean minced (ground) beef
300 g (10½ oz) tinned red kidney beans, rinsed and drained
1 tbsp no-added-salt tomato paste (concentrated purée)

325 g (11½ oz) 99% fat-free mild tomato salsa
extra light sour cream or low-fat yoghurt, to serve

PREP TIME: 20 MINUTES
COOKING TIME: 40 MINUTES
SERVES 4

Preheat the oven to 200°C (400°F/Gas 6). Prick the sweet potatoes a few times with a skewer. Bake on the oven rack for 40 minutes, or until cooked through.

Meanwhile, heat a non-stick frying pan over medium heat. Lightly spray with the oil. Add the garlic and onion and cook for 2–3 minutes, or until softened. Add the beef and cook, breaking up any lumps with a wooden spoon, for 5 minutes, or until browned. Drain off any excess fat. Stir in the kidney beans, tomato paste and salsa. Bring to the boil, then reduce the heat and simmer for 10 minutes, or until slightly thickened.

Make a deep cut along the top of each cooked sweet potato. Divide the mixture among them and top with a dollop of extra-light sour cream or low-fat yoghurt, if you like.

nutrition per serve: Energy 1350 kJ (322 Cal); Fat 5.8 g; Saturated fat 2 g; Protein 21.1 g; Carbohydrate 41.8 g; Fibre 8.5 g; Cholesterol 32 mg

SOUPS AND SALADS

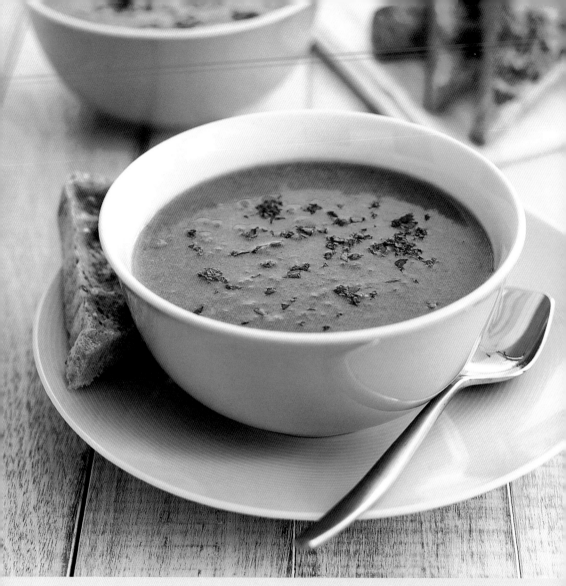

THIS CLASSIC SOUP IS LOW-GI AND LOW-FAT. IT IS ALSO A GOOD SOURCE OF POTASSIUM, BETACAROTENE AND LYCOPENE.

nutrition per serve: Energy 529 kJ (126 Cal)
Fat 3 g
Saturated fat 0.5 g
Protein 7.6 g
Carbohydrate 15.1 g
Fibre 4.1 g
Cholesterol 6 mg

TOMATO SOUP

2 tsp olive or canola oil
1 celery stalk, finely chopped
1 onion, finely chopped
1 carrot, finely chopped
2 garlic cloves, crushed
800 g (1 lb 12 oz) tinned chopped
    tomatoes
750 ml (26 fl oz/3 cups) reduced-salt
    chicken or vegetable stock
1 tbsp no-added-salt tomato paste

1 parsley sprig
1 bay leaf
250 ml (9 fl oz/1 cup) low-fat milk
3 tbsp finely chopped flat-leaf (Italian)
    parsley
wholegrain toast, to serve

PREP TIME: 15 MINUTES
COOKING TIME: 25 MINUTES
SERVES 4

Melt the oil in a saucepan and sauté the celery, onion and carrot for 3–4 minutes. Add the garlic and cook for 30 seconds. Add the chopped tomatoes, chicken or vegetable stock, tomato paste, parsley sprig and bay leaf. Bring to the boil, then simmer for 15 minutes. Remove the parsley and bay leaf.

Purée the soup coarsely in a blender, then return it to the pan. Stir through the milk and heat until hot.

Garnish with the parsley and serve with toasted wholegrain bread.

ROASTED RED CAPSICUM SOUP

ROASTED RED CAPSICUMS AND TOMATOES ARE A GREAT FLAVOUR
COMBINATION AND MAKE THIS VEGETARIAN SOUP A RICH SOURCE OF
THE ANTIOXIDANT BETACAROTENE.

4 large red capsicums (peppers)

4 ripe tomatoes

2 tsp olive or canola oil

1 red onion, chopped

1 garlic clove, crushed

**1 litre (35 fl oz/4 cups) reduced-salt
   vegetable stock**

1 tsp sweet chilli sauce

parmesan cheese, to serve

flat-leaf (Italian) parsley, to serve

6 thick slices wholegrain bread

PREP TIME: 30 MINUTES

COOKING TIME: 45 MINUTES

SERVES 6

Cut the capsicums into large flat pieces, removing the seeds and membrane. Put skin side
up under a hot grill (broiler) until blackened. Leave covered with a tea towel until cool, then
peel away the skin and chop the flesh.

To peel the tomatoes, score a cross in the base of each one. Cover with boiling water for
30 seconds, then plunge into cold water. Drain and peel away the tomato skin from the
cross. Cut in half, scoop out the seeds and roughly chop the flesh.

Heat the oil in a large frying pan and add the onion. Cook over medium heat for
10 minutes, stirring frequently, until very soft. Add the garlic and cook for a further
minute. Add the capsicum, tomato and stock. Bring to the boil, reduce the heat and
simmer for about 20 minutes.

Coarsely purée the soup in a food processor or blender (in batches if necessary). Return
to the pan to reheat gently and stir in the chilli sauce. Top with fresh parsley and shavings
of parmesan cheese. Serve with sliced wholegrain bread.

nutrition per serve: Energy 730 kJ (174 Cal); Fat 3.5 g; Saturated fat 0.5 g; Protein 6.7 g;
Carbohydrate 26.6 g; Fibre 5 g; Cholesterol 0 mg

SPLIT PEA SOUP

A GREAT WAY TO INCLUDE LEGUMES IN YOUR DIET, THIS DELICIOUS LOW-GI SOUP PROVIDES SOLUBLE FIBRE, FOLATE, B-GROUP VITAMINS AND MINERALS.

2 tbsp olive or canola oil
1 large brown onion, chopped
1 large carrot, cut into 1 cm (½ in) cubes
1 large celery stick, cut into 1 cm (½ in) cubes
2 bay leaves
1 tbsp thyme, finely chopped
6 garlic cloves, finely chopped
440 g (15½ oz/2 cups) yellow split peas

1 litre (35 fl oz/4 cups) reduced-salt chicken stock
60 ml (2 fl oz/¼ cup) lemon juice

PREP TIME: 20 MINUTES
COOKING TIME: 1 HOUR 20 MINUTES
SERVES 6–8

Heat the oil in a large saucepan over medium heat. Add the onion, carrot and celery, and cook for 4–5 minutes, or until starting to brown. Add the bay leaves, thyme and garlic and cook for 1 minute.

Stir in the split peas, then add the chicken stock and 1 litre (35 fl oz/4 cups) water. Cook for 1 hour 15 minutes, or until the split peas and vegetables are soft. Stir often during cooking to prevent the soup from sticking to the bottom of the pan, and skim any scum from the surface. Add a little extra water if the soup is too thick.

Remove the soup from the heat and discard the bay leaves. Stir in the lemon juice and season with freshly ground black pepper.

nutrition per serve (8): Energy 988 kJ (236 Cal); Fat 5.9 g; Saturated fat 0.8 g; Protein 14.6 g; Carbohydrate 28.4 g; Fibre 6.5 g; Cholesterol 1 mg

MEDITERRANEAN FISH SOUP

½ tsp saffron threads

2 tsp olive or canola oil

2 large onions, thinly sliced

1 leek, chopped

4 garlic cloves, finely chopped

1 bay leaf, torn

½ tsp dried marjoram

1 tsp grated orange zest

2 tbsp dry white wine (optional)

1 red capsicum (pepper), cut into bite-sized pieces

500 g (1 lb 2 oz) ripe tomatoes, chopped

125 ml (4 fl oz/½ cup) tomato passata (puréed tomatoes) (see Hints)

500 ml (17 fl oz/2 cups) reduced-salt fish or vegetable stock

2 tbsp no-added-salt tomato paste (concentrated purée)

1 tsp soft brown sugar

500 g (1 lb 2 oz) skinless and boneless fish fillets, trimmed and cut into bite-sized pieces (see Hints)

3 tbsp chopped flat-leaf (Italian) parsley

4 wholegrain bread rolls or slices

PREP TIME: 30 MINUTES

COOKING TIME: 45 MINUTES

SERVES 4

Soak the saffron threads in a small bowl with 2 tablespoons of boiling water.

Heat the oil in a large saucepan over low heat. Add the onion, leek, garlic, bay leaf and marjoram. Cover and cook for 10 minutes, shaking the pan occasionally until the onion is soft. Add the zest, wine, capsicum and tomato, cover and cook for 10 minutes.

Add the tomato passata, stock, tomato paste, sugar and saffron (with the liquid) to the pan. Stir well and bring to the boil, then reduce the heat to low and simmer, uncovered, for 15 minutes.

Add the fish to the soup, cover and cook for 8 minutes, or until tender. Add half the parsley, then season with freshly ground black pepper. Discard the bay leaf. Sprinkle the soup with the remaining parsley just before serving.

Warm the bread, then serve with the soup.

HINTS:
• Passata or Italian tomato purée is available in jars at supermarkets.
• Try snapper, red mullet, red rock cod or ocean perch.

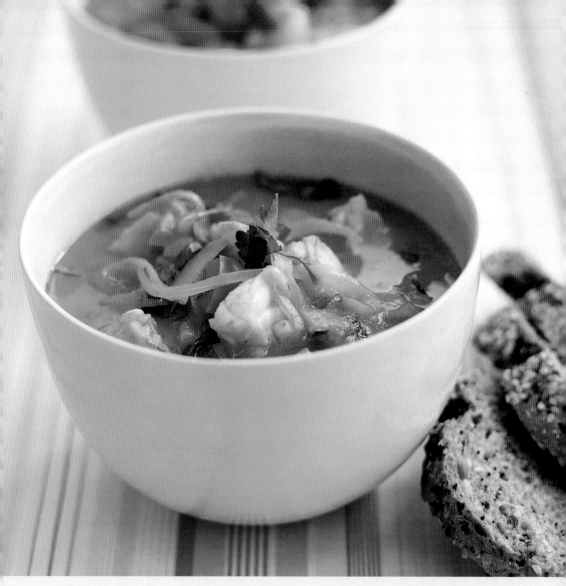

THIS SOUP EVOKES THE WARMTH OF
THE MEDITERRANEAN AND IS A GREAT
WAY TO INCLUDE FISH IN YOUR DIET.
IT'S A GOOD SOURCE OF PROTEIN,
ANTIOXIDANTS, B-GROUP VITAMINS AND
MINERALS, AND IS LOW IN FAT.

nutrition per serve: Energy 1594 kJ (381 Cal)
Fat 6.4 g
Saturated fat 1.1 g
Protein 34.4 g
Carbohydrate 40.2 g
Fibre 8.4 g
Cholesterol 54 mg

COUNTRY-STYLE VEGETABLE SOUP

A SATISFYING LOW-GI MEAL THE WHOLE FAMILY WILL ENJOY, THIS SOUP IS ALSO AN EASY WAY TO INCLUDE LEGUMES AND A VARIETY OF DIFFERENT VEGETABLES IN YOUR DIET.

225 g (8 oz/1 cup) soup mix or pearl barley
2 tsp olive or canola oil
1 leek, thinly sliced
2 garlic cloves, finely chopped
1 green capsicum (pepper), chopped
2 zucchini (courgettes), sliced
2 celery stalks, sliced
125 g (4½ oz) button mushrooms, sliced
2 carrots, sliced
2 orange sweet potatoes, peeled and chopped

2 litres (70 fl oz/8 cups) reduced-salt vegetable stock
175 g (6 oz) broccoli, cut into small florets
1 large handful flat-leaf (Italian) parsley, finely chopped

PREP TIME: 25 MINUTES + OVERNIGHT SOAKING
COOKING TIME: 1 HOUR
SERVES 6

Put the soup mix or barley in a large bowl, cover with water and leave to soak for 8 hours, or overnight. Drain and rinse well.

Heat the oil in a large saucepan and cook the leek and garlic for 5 minutes, or until soft. Add the capsicum, zucchini, celery and mushrooms and cook for 5 minutes, or until starting to become soft. Add the carrot, sweet potato and soup mix and stir well.

Pour in the stock and bring to the boil. Reduce the heat to low, partially cover the pan with a lid and simmer for 45 minutes, or until the vegetables and soup mix are just soft. Add the broccoli florets and cook a further 5 minutes until broccoli is just cooked. Sprinkle with parsley and season with freshly ground black pepper to serve. For a thinner soup add a little water.

HINTS:
• The soup will keep for 2 days in the refrigerator or in the freezer for 1 month. Bring to the boil before serving.
• Soup mix is a combination of pearl barley, split peas and lentils. Both pearl barley and soup mix are readily available from supermarkets.

nutrition per serve: Energy 965 kJ (231 Cal); Fat 3.7 g; Saturated fat 0.7 g; Protein 8.1 g; Carbohydrate 36.7 g; Fibre 11.9 g; Cholesterol 27 mg

BEAN AND SAUSAGE SOUP

SOUP IS A GREAT WAY TO WARM UP ON A COLD WINTER'S NIGHT. THIS ONE IS
RICH AND HEARTY AND WILL SATISFY THE WHOLE FAMILY.

12 tsp olive or canola oil
4 thin low-fat beef sausages
2 leeks, sliced
1 garlic clove, crushed
1 large carrot, chopped into small cubes
2 celery stalks, sliced
2 tbsp plain (all-purpose) flour
2 litres (70 fl oz/8 cups) reduced-salt beef stock

125 ml (4 fl oz/½ cup) white wine (see Hints)
125 g (4½ oz/1½ cups) small pasta shells
400 g (14 oz) tinned three-bean mix, drained and rinsed (see Hints)
1 tsp chopped fresh chilli (optional)

PREP TIME: 25 MINUTES
COOKING TIME: 30 MINUTES
SERVES 4–6

Heat the oil in a large heavy-based saucepan and add the sausages. Cook over medium heat for 5 minutes, or until golden, turning regularly. Drain the cooked sausages on paper towels, and then dice.

Add the leek, garlic, carrot and celery to the pan and cook, stirring occasionally, for 2–3 minutes, or until soft.

Add the flour and cook, stirring, for 1 minute. Add the stock and wine and bring to the boil, then reduce the heat and simmer for 10 minutes.

Add the pasta, beans and chilli (if using) to the pan. Increase the heat and cook for 8–10 minutes, or until the pasta is *al dente*. Return the sausage to the soup and season to taste with freshly ground black pepper. Serve with some low-GI wholegrain bread and a mixed salad for a complete meal.

HINTS:
- If you'd prefer not to use wine, the same amount of liquid can be replaced with reduced-salt beef stock.
- You can use dried beans, if you prefer. Put them in a large bowl, cover with water and leave to soak overnight. Drain and rinse well, then transfer to a large saucepan with enough water to come about 3 cm (1¼ in) above the beans. Bring to a simmer and cook for 1 hour. Drain well before adding to the soup. Boiled dried beans have a slightly lower GI value than tinned beans. They also have a denser texture, making them slightly more filling.

nutrition per serve (6): Energy 962 kJ (230 Cal); Fat 5.3 g; Saturated fat 1.5 g; Protein 11.7 g; Carbohydrate 27.8 g; Fibre 6.1 g; Cholesterol 4 mg

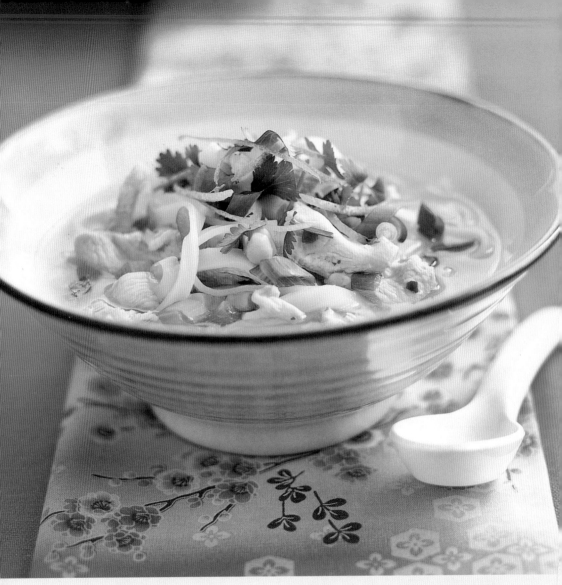

THIS IS A GREAT RECIPE FOR
BUSY PEOPLE—IT CAN BE
PREPARED IN LESS THAN
30 MINUTES IF YOU HAVE ALL
THE INGREDIENTS ON HAND,
GIVING YOU A QUICK, FILLING,
LOW-GI MEAL.

nutrition per serve: Energy 1391 kJ (332 Cal)
Fat 3.1 g
Saturated fat 0.9 g
Protein 33 g
Carbohydrate 40 g
Fibre 3.8 g
Cholesterol 88 mg

THAI-STYLE CHICKEN AND CORN SOUP

1 litre (35 fl oz/4 cups) reduced-salt
  chicken stock
425 g (15 oz) tinned corn kernels,
  undrained
8 spring onions (scallions), sliced
1 tbsp finely chopped fresh ginger
500 g (1 lb 2 oz) lean skinless chicken
  breast, trimmed and thinly sliced
1 tbsp sweet chilli sauce
1 tbsp fish sauce

200 g (7 oz) fresh thin rice noodles
2 large handfuls coriander (cilantro) leaves,
  chopped
2 tsp grated lime zest
2 tbsp lime juice

PREP TIME: 15 MINUTES

COOKING TIME: 10 MINUTES

SERVES 4

Bring the stock to the boil in a large saucepan over high heat. Add the corn kernels and their juice, spring onion and ginger, then reduce the heat and simmer for 1 minute.

Add the chicken, sweet chilli sauce and fish sauce and simmer for 3 minutes, or until the chicken is cooked through.

Put the noodles in a large heatproof bowl, cover with boiling water and soak for 5 minutes, or until softened. Separate gently and drain.

Add the noodles, coriander, lime zest and lime juice to the soup and serve immediately.

MINESTRONE PRIMAVERA

THIS SOUP CELEBRATES THE RETURN OF SPRING WITH A MIX OF FRESH GREEN VEGETABLES. IT IS A GOOD SOURCE OF FIBRE, FOLATE, POTASSIUM AND BETACAROTENE.

1 tbsp olive or canola oil

60 g (2¼ oz) low-fat bacon slices (we used 97% fat-free), finely chopped

2 onions, chopped

2 garlic cloves, thinly sliced

2 small celery stalks, sliced

2 litres (70 fl oz/8 cups) reduced-salt chicken stock

50 g (1¾ oz/⅓ cup) macaroni

2 zucchini (courgettes), chopped

150 g (5½ oz/2 cups) shredded savoy cabbage

150 g (5½ oz/1 cup) frozen peas

175 g (6 oz) green beans, trimmed and chopped

40 g (1½ oz/1 cup) shredded English spinach leaves

400 g (14 oz) tinned cannellini beans, drained and rinsed

1 large handful basil, chopped

grated parmesan cheese, to serve

PREP TIME: 25 MINUTES

COOKING TIME: 40 MINUTES

SERVES 4–6

Heat the oil in a large saucepan. Add the bacon, onion, garlic and celery and cook over low heat for 8 minutes, stirring occasionally until the vegetables are soft but not brown. Add the stock and bring to the boil. Simmer, covered, for 10 minutes.

Add the macaroni and boil for 12 minutes, or until almost *al dente*. Stir in the zucchini, cabbage, peas and beans and simmer for 5 minutes. Add the spinach, cannellini beans and basil and simmer for 2 minutes. Season with freshly ground black pepper and serve with the grated parmesan.

nutrition per serve (6): Energy 822 kJ (196 Cal); Fat 4.3 g; Saturated fat 0.8 g; Protein 14.9 g; Carbohydrate 21.9 g; Fibre 7.6 g; Cholesterol 10 mg

ASPARAGUS AND MUSHROOM SALAD

THIS STYLISH SALAD IS IDEAL AS A STARTER OR AS A SIDE DISH WITH MEAT OR FISH. THE FLAVOURS AND TEXTURES OF THE MUSHROOMS AND ASPARAGUS COMPLEMENT EACH OTHER PERFECTLY.

75 g (6 oz) asparagus, trimmed
1 tbsp wholegrain mustard
1 tbsp grated orange zest
2 tsp grated lemon zest
2 tsp grated lime zest
3 tbsp orange juice
2 tbsp lemon juice
1 tbsp lime juice
2 garlic cloves, crushed
1 tsp sugar

400 g (14 oz) button mushrooms, halved
150 g (5½ oz) rocket (arugula)
1 red capsicum (pepper), cut into strips

PREP TIME: 20 MINUTES
COOKING TIME: 10 MINUTES
SERVES 4

Snap the woody ends from the asparagus spears and cut in half on the diagonal. Cook in boiling water for 1 minute, or until just tender. Drain, plunge into cold water and set aside.

Put the mustard, citrus zest and juice, garlic and sugar in a large saucepan and season with freshly ground black pepper. Bring to the boil, then reduce the heat and add the mushrooms, tossing for 2 minutes. Cool.

Remove the mushrooms from the sauce with a slotted spoon. Return the sauce to the heat, bring to the boil, then reduce the heat and simmer for 3–5 minutes, or until reduced. Cool slightly.

Toss the mushrooms, rocket leaves, capsicum and asparagus together. Put on a plate and drizzle with the sauce.

nutrition per serve: Energy 304 kJ (73 Cal); Fat 0.8 g; Saturated fat 0.01 g; Protein 6.4 g; Carbohydrate 7.1 g; Fibre 4.5 g; Cholesterol 0 mg

WARM PRAWN, ROCKET AND FETA SALAD

1 kg (2 lb 4 oz) raw prawns (shrimp)
4 spring onions (scallions), chopped
4 roma (plum) tomatoes, chopped
1 red capsicum (pepper), chopped
400 g (14 oz) tinned chickpeas, drained and
　rinsed
1 tbsp chopped dill
3 tbsp finely shredded basil
1 tbsp extra virgin olive oil
1 tbsp reduced-fat olive or canola oil
　margarine

2 small fresh red chillies, finely chopped
4 garlic cloves, crushed
2 tbsp lemon juice
300 g (10½ oz) rocket (arugula)
125 g (4½ oz) low-fat feta cheese

PREP TIME: 30 MINUTES
COOKING TIME: 10 MINUTES
SERVES 4–6

Peel the prawns, leaving the tails intact. Gently pull out the dark vein from each prawn back, starting at the head end.

Combine the spring onion, tomato, capsicum, chickpeas and herbs in a bowl and mix well.

Heat the oil and margarine in a large frying pan or wok. Add the prawns and cook, stirring, over high heat for 3 minutes. Add the chilli and garlic, and continue cooking until the prawns turn pink. Remove from the heat and stir in the lemon juice.

Arrange the rocket leaves on a large platter, top with the tomato mixture, then the prawn mixture. Crumble the feta cheese over the top.

HINT:
• If serving as a main meal enjoy this salad with some wholegrain bread or stoneground wholemeal pitta bread, a bean salad or basmati rice.

THIS COLOURFUL LOW-GI
SALAD WILL IMPRESS YOUR
FRIENDS AND FAMILY, AND IS
SUITABLE AS A STARTER OR A
MAIN MEAL.

nutrition per serve (6): Energy 1029 kJ (246 Cal)
Fat 10.5 g
Saturated fat 3 g
Protein 26.7 g
Carbohydrate 9.1 g
Fibre 4 g
Cholesterol 128 mg

SPICY LENTIL SALAD

LENTILS, LIKE ALL LEGUMES, ARE A NATURAL SUPER FOOD—THEY'RE LOW GI, A GREAT SOURCE OF FIBRE, AND PROVIDE GOOD AMOUNTS OF VITAMINS, MINERALS AND ANTIOXIDANTS.

200 g (7 oz/1 cup heaped) basmati rice
185 g (6½ oz/1 cup) brown lentils
1 tsp ground turmeric
1 tsp ground cinnamon
6 cardamom pods
3 star anise
2 bay leaves
3 tbsp olive or canola oil
1 tbsp lemon juice
250 g (9 oz) broccoli florets
2 carrots, peeled and cut into julienne strips
1 onion, finely chopped
2 garlic cloves, crushed
1 red capsicum (pepper), finely chopped

1 tsp garam masala
1 tsp ground coriander
250 g (9 oz/1⅔ cups) fresh or frozen peas, thawed if frozen

DRESSING
250 g (9 oz/1 cup) low-fat plain yoghurt
1 tbsp lemon juice
1 tbsp chopped mint
1 tsp cumin seeds

PREP TIME: 30 MINUTES
COOKING TIME: 1 HOUR 15 MINUTES
SERVES 6

Put the rice, lentils, turmeric, cinnamon, cardamom pods, star anise and bay leaves in a saucepan with 750 ml (26 fl oz/3 cups) of water. Stir well and bring to the boil. Reduce the heat, cover and simmer gently for 50–60 minutes, or until the liquid is absorbed. Remove the whole spices. Transfer the mixture to a large bowl. Whisk 2 tablespoons of the oil with the lemon juice, then fork through the rice mixture.

Steam or boil the broccoli and carrots until tender. Drain and refresh in cold water.

Heat the remaining oil in a large frying pan and add the onion, garlic and capsicum. Stir-fry for 2–3 minutes, then add the garam masala and coriander and stir-fry for a further 1–2 minutes. Add the cooked vegetables and peas and toss to coat in the spice mixture. Add to the rice and fork through to combine. Cover and refrigerate until cold.

To make the dressing, mix the yoghurt, lemon juice, mint and cumin seeds together, then season with freshly ground black pepper. Spoon the salad into six individual bowls or onto a platter and top with the dressing.

nutrition per serve: Energy 1626 kJ (388 Cal); Fat 11.9 g; Saturated fat 2.0 g; Protein 17.1 g; Carbohydrate 48.1 g; Fibre 10.5 g; Cholesterol 7 mg

TUNA, WHITE BEAN AND TOMATO SALAD

READY IN UNDER 30 MINUTES, THIS MEAL IS A GOOD CHOICE FOR A QUICK AND HEALTHY WEEKDAY DINNER. SERVE WITH WHOLEGRAIN BREAD FOR A COMPLETE, SATISFYING MEAL.

3 eggs
850 g (1 lb 14 oz) tinned tuna in spring water, drained
1 garlic clove, crushed
1 tbsp roughly chopped thyme
1 tbsp finely chopped flat-leaf (Italian) parsley
125 ml (4 fl oz/½ cup) fat-free, low-calorie Italian dressing

400 g (14 oz) tinned cannellini beans, drained and rinsed
1 large red onion, coarsely chopped
3 ripe tomatoes, cut into wedges

PREP TIME: 20 MINUTES
COOKING TIME: 5 MINUTES
SERVES 4–6

Fill a saucepan with cold water and gently add the eggs. Bring to the boil, then reduce the heat and simmer for 6 minutes. Drain and plunge the eggs into cold water to stop the cooking process. Peel and cut into wedges.

Drain the tuna and flake into chunks. Combine the garlic, thyme, parsley and dressing in a bowl and whisk with a fork. Season with freshly ground black pepper.

Combine the beans and onion in a large bowl, add the dressing and toss well. Add the tuna, toss gently, then add half the egg wedges and half the tomato. Lightly combine. Pile on a platter and garnish with the remaining egg and tomato.

nutrition per serve (6): Energy 963 kJ (230 Cal); Fat 5.6 g; Saturated fat 1.9 g; Protein 32.9 g; Carbohydrate 9.3 g; Fibre 4.5; Cholesterol 160 mg

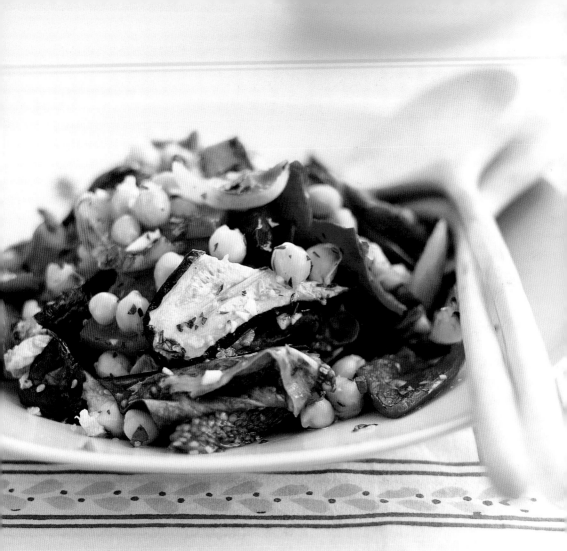

THIS IS A NUTRITIOUS AND
SATISFYING VEGETARIAN MEAL
OR SIDE DISH. IT IS LOW IN FAT
AND RICH IN BETACAROTENE,
FIBRE AND POTASSIUM.

nutrition per serve (6): Energy 752 kJ (180 Cal)

Fat 2.9 g

Saturated fat 0.3 g

Protein 8.4 g

Carbohydrate 25.4 g

Fibre 9 g

Cholesterol 0 mg

CHICKPEA AND ROAST VEGETABLE SALAD

500 g (1 lb 2 oz) orange sweet potato, peeled and cubed
2 red capsicums (peppers), halved and core removed
4 slender eggplants (aubergines), halved lengthways
4 zucchini (courgettes), halved lengthways
4 onions, quartered
olive or canola oil spray
600 g (1 lb 5 oz) tinned chickpeas, drained and rinsed
2 tbsp chopped flat-leaf (Italian) parsley

DRESSING
125 ml (4 fl oz/½ cup) fat-free, low-calorie Italian dressing
1 garlic clove, crushed
1 tbsp chopped thyme

PREP TIME: 25 MINUTES + 30 MINUTES STANDING
COOKING TIME: 40 MINUTES
SERVES 8

Preheat the oven to 220°C (425°F /Gas 7). Line two baking trays with baking paper and lay out the vegetables in a single layer. Lightly spray with oil.

Bake for 40 minutes, or until the vegetables are tender and begin to brown slightly on the edges. Allow to cool. Remove the skins from the capsicum if you like. Chop the capsicum, eggplant and zucchini into pieces, then put the vegetables in a bowl with the chickpeas and half the parsley.

Whisk together the dressing ingredients. Season with freshly ground black pepper, then toss with the vegetables. Leave for 30 minutes, then sprinkle with the rest of the parsley before serving.

WARM MARINATED MUSHROOM SALAD

THIS TASTY SALAD IS A GREAT SIDE DISH AT BARBECUES. IT IS LOW GI AND A GOOD SOURCE OF ANTIOXIDANTS.

750 g (1 lb 9 oz) mixed mushrooms
    (see Hint)
2 garlic cloves, finely chopped
½ tsp green peppercorns, crushed
2 tbsp olive oil
4 tbsp freshly squeezed orange juice
250 g (9 oz) salad leaves, such as lettuce,
    rocket, watercress or baby English
    spinach leaves

olive or canola oil spray
1 tsp finely grated orange zest

PREP TIME: 25 MINUTES + 20 MINUTES
    MARINATING
COOKING TIME: 5 MINUTES
SERVES 4

Trim the mushroom stems and wipe the mushrooms with a damp paper towel. Cut any large mushrooms in half. Mix together the garlic, peppercorns, olive oil and orange juice. Pour over the mushrooms and marinate for about 20 minutes.

Arrange the salad leaves in a dish.

Heat a chargrill pan or barbecue hotplate to hot. Spray with oil. Drain the mushrooms, reserving the marinade. First cook the flat and button mushrooms on the chargrill pan for about 2 minutes. Add the softer mushrooms and cook for 1 minute, or until they just soften.

Scatter the mushrooms over the salad leaves and drizzle with the marinade. Sprinkle with orange zest and season well with freshly ground black pepper.

HINT:
• Try a mix of mushrooms, such as baby button, oyster, Swiss brown, shiitake and enoki.

nutrition per serve: Energy 686 kJ (164 Cal); Fat 10.3 g; Saturated fat 1.4 g; Protein 7.6 g; Carbohydrate 6.6 g; Fibre 6.5 g; Cholesterol 0 mg

SALAD NIÇOISE

THIS COLOURFUL AND NUTRITIOUS SALAD, A MEDITERRANEAN FAVOURITE, IS AN EXCELLENT WAY TO INCLUDE THE NUTRITIONAL BENEFITS OF FISH IN YOUR DIET.

4 eggs

250 g (9 oz) green beans, trimmed

6 artichoke hearts in brine, drained

350 g (12 oz) mixed salad leaves

4 tomatoes, cut into wedges

425 g (15 oz) tinned tuna in spring water, drained and separated into chunks

1 red capsicum (pepper), cut into strips

400 g (14 oz) tinned cannellini beans, drained and rinsed

1 tbsp capers

10 small black olives

1 tbsp chopped tarragon

DRESSING

1 garlic clove, crushed

3 tsp Dijon mustard

2 anchovy fillets in brine, drained and finely chopped

125 ml (4 fl oz/½ cup) fat-free, low-calorie French dressing

PREP TIME: 25 MINUTES

COOKING TIME: 10 MINUTES

SERVES 4–6

Fill a saucepan with cold water and gently add the eggs. Bring to the boil, then reduce the heat and simmer for 6 minutes. Drain and plunge the eggs into cold water to stop the cooking process. Peel and cut into wedges.

Put the beans in a saucepan of boiling water, return to the boil for 2 minutes, then drain and rinse under cold water. Chill in a bowl of iced water. Cut the artichokes into halves or quarters.

Arrange the salad leaves on a platter or individual plates. Top with the green beans, tomato, artichoke, tuna, egg, red capsicum and cannellini beans. Sprinkle with the capers and olives.

To make the dressing, put the garlic, mustard, anchovies and dressing in a bowl and whisk until well blended. Season with freshly ground black pepper and drizzle over the salad. Sprinkle with tarragon.

nutrition per serve (6): Energy 933 kJ (223 Cal); Fat 6.2 g; Saturated fat 1.7 g; Protein 24.8 g; Carbohydrate 12.4 g; Fibre 8.5 g; Cholesterol 170 mg

WARM LAMB SALAD

2 tbsp red curry paste
3 tbsp chopped coriander (cilantro) leaves
1 tbsp finely grated fresh ginger
1 tbsp peanut oil
750 g (1 lb 10 oz) lean lamb loin fillets,
    trimmed and thinly sliced
200 g (7 oz) snow peas (mangetout),
    trimmed
600 g (1 lb 5 oz) thick fresh rice noodles
olive or canola oil spray
1 red capsicum (pepper), thinly sliced
1 Lebanese (short) cucumber, thinly sliced
6 spring onions (scallions), thinly sliced

DRESSING
1 tbsp peanut oil
3 tbsp lime juice
2 tsp soft brown sugar
3 tsp fish sauce
3 tsp reduced-sodium soy sauce
4 tbsp chopped mint leaves
1 garlic clove, crushed

PREP TIME: 30 MINUTES + 3 HOURS
    REFRIGERATION
COOKING TIME: 15 MINUTES
SERVES 4–6

Combine the curry paste, coriander, ginger and peanut oil in a bowl. Add the lamb and coat well. Cover and refrigerate for 2–3 hours.

Steam or boil the snow peas until just tender, then refresh under cold water and drain.

Put the noodles in a large heatproof bowl, cover with boiling water and soak for 8 minutes, or until softened. Separate gently and drain.

To make the dressing, put all the ingredients in a small bowl and whisk until well blended.

Heat a wok until very hot. Spray with the oil. Add half the lamb and stir-fry for 5 minutes, or until tender. Repeat with the remaining lamb, using more spray oil if needed.

Put the lamb, snow peas, noodles, capsicum, cucumber and spring onion in a large bowl, drizzle with the dressing and toss together before serving

HINT:
• This recipe can also be made into a gluten-free version if you use gluten-free fish sauce and gluten-free soy sauce.

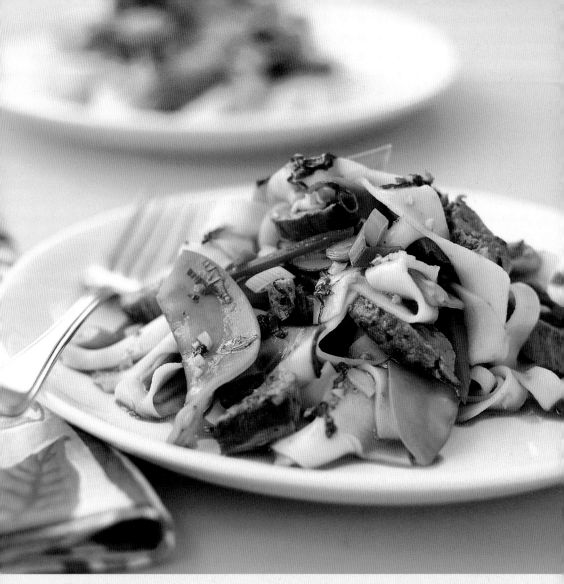

THIS SALAD IS A GOOD
SOURCE OF IRON, ZINC
AND ANTIOXIDANTS.

nutrition per serve (6): Energy 1822 kJ (435 Cal)

Fat 12.6 g

Saturated fat 3.2 g

Protein 31.8 g

Carbohydrate 46.2 g

Fibre 3 g

Cholesterol 81 mg

TOFU SALAD WITH GINGER MISO DRESSING

THIS ASIAN-THEMED SALAD IS A DELICIOUS LIGHT VEGETARIAN MEAL OR SIDE DISH. SERVE WITH FRESH RICE NOODLES OR BASMATI RICE.

4½ tbsp tamari (see Hint)

1 tsp olive or canola oil

2 garlic cloves, crushed

1 tsp grated fresh ginger

1 tsp chilli paste

500 g (1 lb 2 oz) firm tofu, cut into small cubes

400 g (14 oz) mixed Asian salad leaves

1 Lebanese (short) cucumber, thinly sliced

250 g (9 oz) cherry tomatoes, halved

olive or canola oil spray

DRESSING

2 tsp white miso paste

2 tbsp mirin

1 tsp sesame oil

1 tsp grated fresh ginger

1 tsp finely chopped chives

1 tbsp sesame seeds, toasted

PREP TIME: 20 MINUTES + 10 MINUTES MARINATING

COOKING TIME: 5 MINUTES

SERVES 4

Mix together the tamari, oil, garlic, ginger and chilli paste in a bowl. Add the tofu and mix well. Marinate for 10 minutes. Drain, reserving the marinade.

Put the salad leaves, cucumber and tomato in a bowl.

To make the dressing, combine the miso with 125 ml (4 fl oz/½ cup) hot water and leave until the miso dissolves. Add the mirin, sesame oil, ginger, chives and sesame seeds and stir until it begins to thicken.

Heat a chargrill pan or barbecue hotplate to hot. Spray with oil. Add the tofu and cook over medium heat for 4 minutes, or until golden brown. Increase the heat to high, pour on the reserved marinade and cook for a further 1 minute over high heat. Cool for 5 minutes.

Add the tofu to the salad, drizzle with the dressing and toss well.

HINT:
• Tamari is a naturally fermented, thick, dark Japanese soy sauce. You can use reduced-sodium soy sauce instead.

nutrition per serve: Energy 1069 kJ (255 Cal); Fat 13.2 g; Saturated fat 1.9 g; Protein 19.8 g; Carbohydrate 11.2 g; Fibre 6.2 g; Cholesterol 0 mg

TABOULEH

THIS POPULAR SALAD IS VERY VERSATILE—SERVE IT WITH MEAT OR FISH,
USE IT IN A SANDWICH OR EAT IT ON ITS OWN. IF YOU LIKE TO EXPERIMENT,
LOOK FOR CRACKED BARLEY IN HEALTH FOOD SHOPS TO USE AS A
SUBSTITUTE FOR THE BURGHUL.

125 g (4½ oz/¾ cup) burghul (bulgur)
300 g (10½ oz) flat-leaf (Italian) parsley
1 handful mint leaves
4 spring onions (scallions), finely chopped
4 tomatoes, finely chopped
2 garlic cloves, crushed
3 tbsp lemon juice
2 tbsp olive oil

PREP TIME: 20 MINUTES + 15 MINUTES
STANDING
COOKING TIME: NIL
SERVES 6–8

Put the burghul in a bowl with 185 ml (6 fl oz/3¼ cup) of water and leave for 15 minutes, or until all the water has been absorbed.

Finely chop the herbs with a large sharp knife or in a food processor. Take care not to over-process.

Put the burghul, herbs, spring onion, tomato, garlic, lemon juice and oil in a bowl and toss well. Refrigerate until required. Return to room temperature to serve.

nutrition per serve (8): Energy 504 kJ (120 Cal); Fat 5 g; Saturated fat 0.7 g; Protein 3.7 g; Carbohydrate 11.4 g; Fibre 6.0 g; Cholesterol 0 mg

A LOW-GI DISH WITH A TANGY
FLAVOUR, THIS SALAD
PROVIDES ANTIOXIDANTS,
FOLATE, IRON AND ZINC—
SUITABLE AS A LIGHT MEAL OR
A QUICKLY PREPARED DINNER.

nutrition per serve: Energy 1752 kJ (418 Cal)
Fat 7.4 g
Saturated fat 2.6 g
Protein 34.1 g
Carbohydrate 50.6 g
Fibre 3.7 g
Cholesterol 80 mg

MINTY BEEF NOODLE SALAD

olive or canola oil spray

500 g (1 lb 2 oz) piece lean beef rump steak

250 g (9 oz) dry thin rice vermicelli noodles

250 g (9 oz) cherry tomatoes, halved

200 g (7 oz) baby Asian salad leaves

1 Lebanese (short) cucumber, peeled, seeded and thinly sliced

¼ red onion, cut into thin slivers

6 radishes, thinly sliced

1 handful mint

DRESSING

3 tbsp lime juice

3 tbsp reduced-sodium soy sauce

2 tbsp fish sauce

2 tbsp grated palm sugar or soft brown sugar

2 small red chillies, seeded and finely chopped

PREP TIME: 20 MINUTES

COOKING TIME: 10 MINUTES

SERVES 4

Heat a large, non-stick frying pan and spray with the oil. Pat the meat dry with paper towels. Season well with freshly ground black pepper. Put the meat in the pan and brown on both sides. Cook for a further 5–8 minutes, or until cooked as desired. Cover with foil and set aside for 5 minutes, then cut into thin slices.

Combine the dressing ingredients in a small bowl, stirring to dissolve the sugar.

Cover the noodles with boiling water and set aside for 5 minutes, or until softened. Drain and cool. Use scissors to cut into smaller lengths.

Combine the cherry tomatoes, salad greens, cucumber, onion, radishes and mint leaves in a large bowl. Toss through the noodles and beef, then pour over the dressing.

SPICY THAI PORK SALAD

THIS SPICY SALAD GETS TOP MARKS FOR GOOD TASTE AND HAS THE ADDED BENEFITS OF BEING HEART HEALTHY AND QUICK TO MAKE. SERVE WITH FRESH RICE NOODLES, MUNG BEAN NOODLES OR BASMATI RICE FOR A COMPLETE LOW-GI MEAL.

50 g (1¾ oz/⅓ cup) raw unsalted peanuts

2 tsp olive or canola oil

2 stems lemon grass, white part only, thinly sliced

2 green chillies, finely chopped

500 g (1 lb 2 oz) lean minced (ground) pork

2 tsp finely grated lime zest

3 tbsp lime juice

2–6 tsp chilli sauce

lettuce leaves, to serve

1 handful coriander (cilantro) leaves

1 small handful small mint leaves

1 small onion, very finely sliced

3 tbsp chopped fresh shallots

PREP TIME: 20 MINUTES

COOKING TIME: 10 MINUTES

SERVES 4–6

Preheat the oven to 180°C (350°F/Gas 4). Put the peanuts on a baking tray. Cook for 5 minutes, stirring once, until the peanuts are lightly golden. Cool then chop.

Heat a wok until very hot, add the oil and swirl to coat. Add the lemon grass, chilli and pork. Stir-fry, breaking up any lumps with a fork or wooden spoon, over high heat for 6 minutes, or until cooked through. Transfer to a bowl and set aside to cool completely.

Add the lime zest, lime juice, and the chilli sauce to taste, to the cooled pork mixture. Arrange the lettuce leaves on a plate. Stir most of the coriander and mint leaves, onion, peanuts and shallots through the pork mixture. Spoon over the lettuce and sprinkle the rest of the mint leaves, onion, peanuts and shallots over the top to serve.

nutrition per serve (6): Energy 914 kJ (195 Cal); Fat 11.5 g; Saturated fat 2.9 g; Protein 19.2 g; Carbohydrate 2.7 g; Fibre 1.3 g; Cholesterol 50 mg

HOT BEAN SALAD

A SATISFYING COMBINATION OF HIGH-FIBRE BEANS AND NUTRITIOUS
VEGETABLES AND HERBS, RICH IN SLOW-RELEASE CARBOHYDRATE AND
SOLUBLE FIBRE, THIS SALAD IS IDEAL IF YOU ARE WATCHING YOUR BLOOD
SUGAR AND CHOLESTEROL LEVELS.

100 g (3½ oz) dried chickpeas
100 g (3½ oz) dried pinto beans
100 g (3½ oz) dried red kidney beans
100 g (3½ oz) dried black-eyed beans
1 tbsp olive or canola oil
2 onions, sliced
2 tsp ground cumin
1 tsp ground coriander
420 g (15 oz) tinned corn kernels, drained
2 tomatoes, chopped

4 tbsp lemon juice
1 large handful coriander (cilantro) leaves,
  chopped
1 Lebanese (short) cucumber, grated
250 g (9 oz/1 cup) low-fat plain yoghurt

PREP TIME: 15 MINUTES + OVERNIGHT
  SOAKING
COOKING TIME: 1 HOUR 15 MINUTES
SERVES 8

Combine the chickpeas, pinto beans, red kidney beans and black-eyed beans in a large
bowl. Cover with water and soak overnight. Drain, place in a large saucepan and cover
with water. Bring to the boil, then reduce the heat and simmer for 45 minutes, or until
tender. Don't overcook or the beans will be mushy.

Meanwhile, in a large, deep non-stick frying pan, heat the oil and then add the onion. Cook
over low heat for 25 minutes, or until golden. Add the cumin and coriander with the beans,
and toss to combine. Add the corn kernels, tomato, lemon juice and coriander. Season
with freshly ground black pepper and stir.

Squeeze out the moisture from the cucumber. Combine the cucumber with the yoghurt,
and season. Stir to combine.

Put the hot bean mixture on a serving plate, and top with the yoghurt mixture.

nutrition per serve: Energy 961 kJ (229 Cal); Fat 2.3 g; Saturated fat 0.3 g; Protein 14.7 g;
Carbohydrate 31.7 g; Fibre 11.4 g; Cholesterol 2 mg

MAIN MEALS

TOFU WITH GREENS AND NOODLES

MARINADE
3 tbsp oyster sauce
3 tbsp hoisin sauce
2 tbsp reduced-sodium soy sauce
1½ tbsp soft brown sugar
3 tsp grated ginger
3 garlic cloves, crushed

300 g (10½ oz) firm tofu, drained and
    cut into 2 cm (¾ in) cubes
300 g (10½ oz) dried thin egg noodles
1 tsp olive or canola oil
4 Asian shallots, thinly sliced

1 small red capsicum (pepper), seeded and
    thinly sliced
200 g (7 oz) sugar snap peas, trimmed
400 g (14 oz) broccolini, cut into 5 cm (2 in)
    lengths (see Hint)
125 ml (4 fl oz/½ cup) reduced-salt
    vegetable stock
coriander (cilantro) leaves, to serve

PREP TIME: 15 MINUTES + 30 MINUTES
    MARINATING
COOKING TIME: 15 MINUTES
SERVES 4

Combine the marinade ingredients in a non-metallic bowl. Add the tofu and gently stir through. Cover and refrigerate for at least 30 minutes, longer if possible.

Cook the noodles according to the manufacturer's directions and drain. Cut the noodles into shorter lengths using scissors.

Heat the oil in a large wok. Add the shallots and capsicum and stir-fry for 2 minutes, or until slightly softened. Add the peas, broccolini and stock. Cover and cook for 2–3 minutes, or until the vegetables are just tender, stirring occasionally.

Add the tofu with the marinade ingredients and the noodles. Gently combine and stir until heated through. Serve immediately garnished with the coriander leaves.

HINT:
• Use broccoli florets if broccolini is not available.

IF YOU THINK TOFU IS BLAND,
WAIT TILL YOU'VE TRIED THIS
DISH. WHEN MARINATED,
THE TOFU SOAKS UP ALL THE
FLAVOURS. THIS DISH IS A GOOD
SOURCE OF ANTIOXIDANTS,
FOLATE, FIBRE AND IRON.

nutrition per serve: Energy 2125 kJ (508 Cal)

Fat 9 g

Saturated fat 1.3 g

Protein 26.4 g

Carbohydrate 73.2 g

Fibre 11.1 g

Cholesterol 14 mg

THAI CHICKEN AND HOLY BASIL STIR-FRY

THIS LOW-GI AROMATIC THAI MEAL PROVIDES GOOD AMOUNTS OF MOST VITAMINS AND MINERALS. THE FRESH FLAVOURS ARE PERFECT TO ENJOY ON A SUMMER NIGHT.

400 g (14 oz) fresh rice noodles

3 tbsp fish sauce

3 tbsp lime juice

1 tomato, diced

2 handfuls Thai (holy) basil

500 g (1 lb 2 oz) skinless chicken breast
   fillets

2 tsp olive or canola oil

3 garlic cloves, thinly sliced

4 spring onions (scallions), thinly sliced

2 small red chillies, seeded and thinly
   sliced

250 g (9 oz) snow peas (mangetout),
   trimmed

PREP TIME: 15 MINUTES

COOKING TIME: 20 MINUTES

SERVES 4

Put the rice noodles in a large heatproof bowl. Cover with boiling water and soak for 8 minutes, or until softened. Seperate gently and drain. Use scissors to cut into shorter lengths.

Meanwhile, to make the stir-fry sauce, put the fish sauce, lime juice, tomato, basil and 1 tablespoon water in a small bowl and mix well.

Trim the chicken and thinly slice. Heat a wok over high heat, add the oil and swirl to coat. Add the garlic, spring onion and chilli and stir-fry for 1 minute, or until fragrant. Add the chicken in small batches and stir-fry for 3 minutes, or until lightly browned. Remove from the wok and set aside. Reheat the wok between batches.

Return all the chicken to the wok. Add the snow peas and stir-fry sauce to the wok and scrape any sediment from the bottom. Stir through the noodles. Reduce the heat and simmer for 2 minutes, or until the tomato is soft and the chicken cooked through. Serve immediately.

nutrition per serve: Energy 1807 kJ (432 Cal); Fat 10.3 g; Saturated fat 2.3 g; Protein 34.8 g; Carbohydrate 46.7 g; Fibre 4.1 g; Cholesterol 82 mg

TERIYAKI PORK WITH STEAMED ASIAN GREENS

THIS POPULAR ASIAN DISH IS LOW IN FAT AND A RICH SOURCE OF PROTEIN, ANTIOXIDANTS, FOLATE AND POTASSIUM.

500 g (1 lb 2 oz) lean pork fillet
125 ml (4 fl oz/½ cup) reduced-sodium soy sauce
125 ml (4 fl oz/½ cup) mirin
125 ml (4 fl oz/½ cup) unsweetened apple juice
1 tbsp grated ginger
3 cm x 3 cm (1¼ in x 1¼ in) piece ginger, sliced
300 g (10½ oz) gai larn (Chinese broccoli), cut into 10 cm (4 in) lengths
200 g (7 oz) asparagus, trimmed and cut into 5 cm (2 in) pieces

115 g (4 oz) fresh baby corn, trimmed
1 tsp sesame oil
olive or canola oil spray
basmati or doongara rice, to serve (see Hint)

PREP TIME: 20 MINUTES + 1 HOUR MARINATING
COOKING TIME: 20 MINUTES
SERVES 4

Thinly slice the pork across the grain. Mix the soy, mirin, apple juice and ginger in a large, non-metallic bowl. Add the pork and toss to coat well. Cover and refrigerate for 1 hour.

Meanwhile, fill a wok one-third full of water, and bring to a simmer over a low heat. Line the base of a bamboo steamer with the ginger slices and top with the gai larn, asparagus and corn. Cover with the lid, place over the wok, making sure the water doesn't touch the base, and steam for 5–6 minutes, or until the vegetables are just cooked. Discard the ginger, drizzle with the sesame oil and season with pepper.

At the same time, lightly spray a non-stick wok with oil and heat over a high heat. Add the pork in two batches and cook for 2–3 minutes, or until cooked. Set aside. Add the marinade and simmer for 4–5 minutes, or until reduced and thickened. Return the pork and stir until warmed through. Serve with the steamed vegetables and rice.

HINT:
• The rice will add a lot more carbohydrate, so if you have difficulty controlling your blood sugar level make sure that you have no more than 1 cup of cooked rice.

nutrition per serve: Energy 1238 kJ (296 Cal); Fat 5.1 g; Saturated fat 1.2 g; Protein 33.1 g; Carbohydrate 23.8 g; Fibre 4.5 g; Cholesterol 119 mg

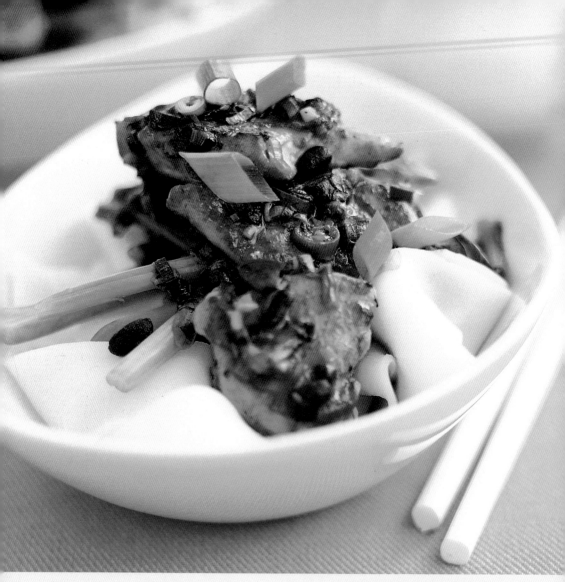

THIS LOW-GI, HIGH-PROTEIN DISH IS A GOOD SOURCE OF B-GROUP VITAMINS, POTASSIUM AND PHOSPHORUS. IT'S A GREAT CHOICE FOR THOSE WATCHING THEIR WEIGHT.

nutrition per serve: Energy 1708 kJ (408 Cal)

Fat 6.2 g

Saturated fat 1.1 g

Protein 49.1 g

Carbohydrate 45.7 g

Fibre 4.9 g

Cholesterol 83 mg

RICE NOODLES WITH FISH AND BLACK BEANS

400 g (14 oz) fresh rice noodles
200 g (7 oz) Chinese broccoli (gai larn),
   cut into 5 cm (2 in) lengths
2 tbsp reduced-sodium soy sauce
1½ tbsp Chinese rice wine (optional)
½ tsp sesame oil
1 tsp cornflour (cornstarch)
550 g (1 lb 4 oz) skinless snapper or
   blue eye fillets
2 tsp olive or canola oil
5 garlic cloves, crushed
2 tsp finely chopped ginger

2 spring onions (scallions), finely chopped,
   plus extra, thinly sliced on the diagonal,
   to garnish
2 small red chillies, finely chopped
2 tbsp tinned salted black beans, rinsed,
   roughly chopped
170 ml (5½ fl oz/⅔ cup) reduced-salt fish
   or vegetable stock

PREP TIME: 20 MINUTES

COOKING TIME: 20 MINUTES

SERVES 4

Put the noodles in a large heatproof bowl, cover with boiling water and soak for 8 minutes, or until softened. Separate gently and drain.

Put the Chinese broccoli in a steamer, cover and steam over a wok or large saucepan of simmering water for 2 minutes, or until slightly wilted. Remove from the heat and keep warm.

To make the marinade, combine the soy sauce, rice wine, sesame oil and cornflour in a large non-metallic bowl. Cut the fish into 4 cm (1½ in) pieces, checking for bones. Add to the marinade and toss to coat well.

Heat a wok over high heat, add the oil and swirl to coat. Add the garlic, ginger, spring onion, chilli and black beans and stir-fry for 1 minute. Add the fish and marinade and cook for 2 minutes, or until the fish is almost cooked through. Remove the fish with a slotted spoon and keep warm. Add the stock to the wok and bring to the boil. Reduce the heat to low and bring to a simmer. Cook for 5 minutes, or until the sauce has slightly thickened. Return the fish to the wok, cover with a lid and simmer gently for 2–3 minutes, or until just cooked.

Divide the noodles among four plates, top with the Chinese broccoli and spoon the fish and black bean sauce on top. Garnish with the extra spring onion.

BEEF SKEWERS WITH TOMATO MINT SALAD

THIS MEAL IS QUICK AND EASY TO MAKE AND IS LOADED WITH FOLATE, POTASSIUM AND ANTIOXIDANTS.

600 g (1 lb 5 oz) lean beef sirloin steaks
1 large red capsicum (pepper)
8 x 4 cm (1¾ in) flat or button mushrooms

MARINADE
3 tbsp reduced-salt teriyaki sauce
1 tbsp pure yellow box honey
1 tbsp lemon juice
2 garlic cloves, crushed

TOMATO MINT SALAD
4 vine-ripened tomatoes, seeded and
  chopped
3 spring onions (scallions), chopped

1 Lebanese (short) cucumber, seeded and
  chopped
2 handfuls mint, chopped
2 tbsp fat-free, low-calorie Italian dressing

olive or canola oil spray
1 tbsp sesame seeds, toasted
basmati or doongara rice, to serve
  (see Hint)

PREP TIME: 25 MINUTES + SOAKING AND
  MARINATING TIME
COOKING TIME: 25 MINUTES
SERVES 4

Soak 8 long wooden skewers in water for 15 minutes. Cut the meat into bite-sized cubes. Seed the capsicum, then cut into 24 x 3 cm (1¼ in) cubes. Thread the meat onto the skewers, alternating with the mushrooms and capsicum.

Combine the marinade ingredients in a non-metallic flat dish. Lay the skewers in the marinade and coat well. Refrigerate for at least 20 minutes, turning occasionally.

Combine the tomato mint salad ingredients in a bowl.

Meanwhile, preheat a grill (broiler) or barbecue. Cook the mainated skewers, turning and spraying lightly with the oil, for 8 minutes, or until just cooked. Brush 2 or 3 times with the remaining marinade. Scatter over the sesame seeds. Serve the skewers with the tomato mint salad and rice.

HINT:
• The rice will add a lot more carbohydrate, so if you have difficulty controlling your blood sugar level make sure that you have no more than 1 cup of cooked rice.

nutrition per serve: Energy 1403 kJ (335 Cal); Fat 12.3 g; Saturated fat 4.4 g; Protein 37.6 g; Carbohydrate 15.3 g; Fibre 5.5 g; Cholesterol 87 mg

FRIED RICE

A REDUCED-FAT FRIED RICE, THIS VERSION IS HIGH IN PROTEIN AND
CARBOHYDRATE, WITH GOOD AMOUNTS OF VITAMIN C, B-GROUP VITAMINS,
POTASSIUM AND PHOSPHORUS.

olive or canola oil spray
4 egg whites, lightly beaten
2 garlic cloves, crushed
350 g (12 oz) raw prawns (shrimp), peeled,
    deveined and halved lengthways
100 g (3½ oz) cooked skinless chicken,
    shredded
80 g (2¾ oz/½ cup) frozen peas
180 g (6½ oz) sliced light ham, cut into
    small strips
1 red capsicum (pepper), diced

4 spring onions (scallions), sliced
750 g (1 lb 10 oz/4 cups) cooked basmati
    or basmati wild rice (see Hint)
1½ tbsp sodium-reduced soy sauce
3 tsp fish sauce
1½ tsp soft brown sugar

PREP TIME: 20 MINUTES
COOKING TIME: 15 MINUTES
SERVES 6

Lightly spray a non-stick wok with oil and pour in the egg white. Cook over low heat,
stirring until the egg is just cooked and slightly scrambled, then remove and set aside.

Add the garlic, prawns, chicken, peas, ham and capsicum to the wok, and stir-fry for
3–4 minutes, or until the prawns are cooked.

Add the spring onion, rice, soy sauce, fish sauce and sugar, and toss for 30 seconds, or
until heated through. Add the egg, toss lightly and serve.

HINT:
• You will need to cook 260 g (9¼ oz/1⅓ cups) rice blend for this recipe.

nutrition per serve: Energy 1225 kJ (293 Cal); Fat 3.4 g; Saturated fat 0.9 g; Protein 24.6 g;
Carbohydrate 38.2 g; Fibre 1.8 g; Cholesterol 85 mg

SPICY CHICKEN STIR-FRY

4 dried shiitake mushrooms

250 g (9 oz) fresh rice noodles or dried
mung bean noodles

olive or canola oil spray

1 red onion, cut into thin wedges

2 garlic cloves, crushed

2 cm x 2 cm (¾ in x ¾ in) piece fresh
ginger, julienned

1 tbsp chilli jam

400 g (14 oz) skinless chicken breast fillet,
cut into strips

½ red capsicum (pepper), cut into thin
strips

800 g (1 lb 12 oz) Chinese broccoli (gai
larn), cut into 5 cm (2 in) lengths

115 g (4 oz) fresh or tinned baby corn,
halved on the diagonal

150 g (5½ oz/1½ cups) snowpeas
(mangetout), halved on the diagonal

4 tbsp reduced-sodium soy sauce

2 tbsp mirin

1 large handful coriander (cilantro) leaves

PREP TIME: 20 MINUTES + 15 MINUTES
SOAKING

COOKING TIME: 15 MINUTES

SERVES 4

Place the mushrooms in a heatproof bowl and cover with 375 ml (13 fl oz/1½ cups) boiling water and stand for 15 minutes. Drain, reserving the liquid and squeezing out any excess liquid. Remove the stalks and thinly slice the caps. Place the noodles in a heatproof bowl, pour over boiling water to cover and stand for 5 minutes, or until tender. Drain.

Meanwhile, heat a non-stick wok over a high heat and spray with the oil. Add the onion and cook for 2–3 minutes. Add the garlic, ginger and chilli jam and cook for a further 1 minute, adding 1–2 tablespoons of the reserved mushroom liquid to mix in the chilli jam.

Add the chicken and cook for 4–5 minutes, or until almost cooked through. Add the capsicum, gai larn, corn, snowpeas, mushrooms and 3 tablespoons reserved mushroom liquid and stir-fry for 2–3 minutes, or until the vegetables are tender. Add the soy sauce, mirin, coriander and noodles and season with ground white pepper. Toss until well combined and serve immediately.

HINT:
• Dried shiitake mushrooms, chilli jam and mirin are readily available in supermarkets and Asian food stores.

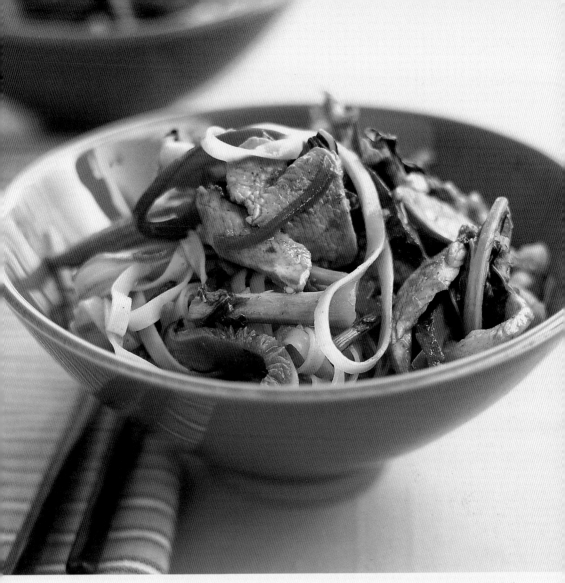

STIR-FRIES ARE AN EASY WAY
TO INCLUDE MORE VEGETABLES
IN YOUR DIET. THIS PEPPED-UP,
TASTY DISH OFFERS GOOD
AMOUNTS OF ANTIOXIDANTS,
B-GROUP VITAMINS AND IRON.

nutrition per serve: Energy 1505 kJ (360 Cal)

Fat 7.3 g

Saturated fat 1.8 g

Protein 32.2 g

Carbohydrate 34.8 g

Fibre 11.3 g

Cholesterol 66 mg

STIR-FRIED THAI BEEF

APART FROM THE MARINATING TIME, THIS DISH IS QUICK TO MAKE, AND IS A GOOD CHOICE FOR BUSY PEOPLE. IT CONTAINS ANTIOXIDANTS, FOLATE, IRON AND ZINC.

400 g (14 oz) lean sirloin steak, trimmed
2–3 bird's eye chillies, seeded and finely chopped
3 garlic cloves, crushed
1 tsp palm sugar or soft brown sugar
2 tbsp fish sauce
2 tsp olive or canola oil
150 g (5½ oz) snake (yard-long) beans, sliced into 3 cm (1¼ in) lengths
150 g (5½ oz) sugar snap peas, trimmed
1 large carrot, thinly sliced

1 large handful Thai basil
1–2 bird's eye chillies, seeded and finely sliced (optional), to garnish
basmati or doongara rice, to serve (see Hints)

PREP TIME: 15 MINUTES + 2 HOURS MARINATING
COOKING TIME: 25 MINUTES
SERVES 4

Slice the meat as thinly as possible, cutting across the grain. Place in a non-metallic bowl with the chilli, garlic, palm sugar, fish sauce and 1 teaspoon of the oil. Toss well to combine, cover and refrigerate for 2 hours.

Blanch the beans, sugar snap peas and carrot in a large saucepan of boiling water for 2 minutes, drain and refresh. Heat the remaining oil in a large, non-stick wok until very hot and stir-fry the beef in 2 batches over high heat until just browned.

Return all the beef to the wok with the blanched vegetables and basil. Stir-fry for a further 1–2 minutes, or until warmed through. Garnish with sliced chillies, if you like, and serve with the rice.

HINTS:
- To save time in the evening, you can prepare the meat in the morning and leave it in the fridge to marinate during the day.
- The rice will add a lot more carbohydrate, so if you have difficulty controlling your blood sugar level make sure that you have no more than 1 cup of cooked rice.

nutrition per serve: Energy 882 kJ (211 Cal); Fat 8.9 g; Saturated fat 2.9 g; Protein 24.4 g; Carbohydrate 5.8 g; Fibre 4.2 g; Cholesterol 58 mg

TANDOORI PORK KEBABS

THE INDIAN SPICES BLEND BEAUTIFULLY WITH THE PORK TO PRODUCE A
MEAL THAT'S RICH IN FLAVOUR. THIS DISH IS A GOOD SOURCE OF PROTEIN,
POTASSIUM AND PHOSPHORUS.

250 g (9 oz/1 cup) low-fat plain yoghurt
2 garlic cloves, crushed
2 tbsp tandoori paste
1 tbsp lemon juice
2 tbsp chopped coriander (cilantro) leaves
600 g (1 lb 5 oz) lean pork fillet, cubed
1 tsp olive or canola oil
1 onion, chopped
2 garlic cloves, crushed, extra
2 tsp ground cumin
½ tsp paprika
1 tsp ground coriander

400 g (14 oz/2 cups) basmati rice
1 litre (35 fl oz/4 cups) reduced-salt
vegetable stock
185 g (6¼ oz/¾ cup) low-fat plain yoghurt,
extra
1 tbsp chopped coriander (cilantro) leaves,
extra

PREP TIME: 20 MINUTES + 4 HOURS
MARINATING
COOKING TIME: 40 MINUTES
SERVES 4

Combine the yoghurt, garlic, tandoori paste, lemon juice and coriander in a large, non-metallic bowl. Add the pork and stir to coat. Refrigerate, covered, for 4 hours.

Heat the oil in a heavy-based saucepan, add the onion, garlic, spices and coriander and cook for 5 minutes, or until golden. Add the rice and stir to coat. Add the stock, bring to the boil, then simmer for 10 minutes, or until tunnels appear in the rice. Reduce the heat to low, cover and cook for 10 minutes.

Thread the pork onto 8 skewers. Heat a chargrill plate and cook for 3–5 minutes on each side, or until tender.

Combine the extra yoghurt and coriander and serve with the pork and spiced rice. Serve with a salad.

HINT:
• Marinate the pork in the morning before work, then cook when you get home.

nutrition per serve: Energy 2652 kJ (634 Cal); Fat 6.8 g; Saturated fat 1.9 g; Protein 48 g; Carbohydrate 91.5 g; Fibre 4.6 g; Cholesterol 168 mg

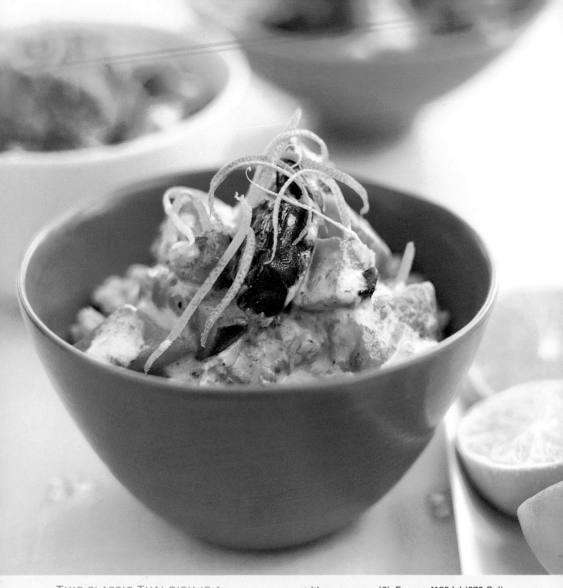

THIS CLASSIC THAI DISH IS A GREAT CHOICE FOR WEIGHT WATCHERS. IT IS A FILLING VEGETARIAN MEAL, AND MAKES DELICIOUS LEFTOVERS.

nutrition per serve (6): Energy 1139 kJ (272 Cal)
Fat 6.9 g
Saturated fat 3.2 g
Protein 6.2 g
Carbohydrate 42.3 g
Fibre 9.2 g
Cholesterol 0 mg

GREEN VEGETABLE CURRY WITH BARLEY

300 g (10½ oz/1½ cups) pearl barley
2 tsp olive or canola oil
1 onion, chopped
1–2 tbsp green curry paste
1 eggplant (aubergine), cut into quarters and sliced
375 ml (13 fl oz/1½ cups) light coconut milk
250 ml (9 fl oz/1 cup) reduced-salt vegetable stock
6 makrut (kaffir lime) leaves

1 sweet potato, peeled and cut into cubes
1 tsp soft brown sugar
2 tbsp lime juice
2 tsp grated lime zest
basmati or doongar rice, to serve (see Hints)

PREP TIME: 15 MINUTES
COOKING TIME: 55 MINUTES
SERVES 4–6

Rinse and drain the barley. Put in a large saucepan with 1.25 litres (44 fl oz/5 cups) water. Bring to the boil, then reduce the heat and simmer for 25–30 minutes, or until tender. Drain.

Meanwhile, heat the oil in a large wok or frying pan. Add the onion and curry paste and cook, stirring, over medium heat for 3 minutes. Add the eggplant and cook for a further 4–5 minutes, or until softened.

Pour in the coconut milk and stock, bring to the boil, then reduce the heat and simmer for 5 minutes. Add the kaffir lime leaves and sweet potato and cook for 10 minutes, or until the eggplant and sweet potato are very tender.

Mix in the sugar, lime juice and lime zest until well combined with the vegetables. Season to taste with freshly ground black pepper and serve with the barley.

HINTS:
- Strict vegetarians should be sure to read the label and choose a green curry paste that doesn't contain shrimp paste. Alternatively, make your own curry pastes.
- The rice will add more carbohydrate, so choose a small serve.

LAMB KEBABS, RAITA AND BULGUR SALAD

NOT ONLY DOES THIS MEAL TASTE DELICIOUS, IT IS ALSO RICH IN CARBOHYDRATE AND PROTEIN AND IS A GOOD SOURCE OF MANY VITAMINS AND MINERALS.

LAMB KEBABS
750 g (1 lb 10 oz) lean lamb
1 tbsp Moroccan seasoning
2 tsp lemon juice
2 garlic cloves, crushed

RAITA
375 g (13 oz/1½ cups) low-fat plain yoghurt
1 small Lebanese (short) cucumber, peeled, seeded and diced
1 large handful mint, chopped

BULGUR SALAD
350 g (12 oz/2 cups) bulgur wheat
125 g (4½ oz) cherry tomatoes, halved

1 large handful flat-leaf (Italian) parsley, chopped
4 tbsp chopped mint
75 g (2½ oz/½ cup) currants
95 g (3¾ oz/½ cup) dried apricots, chopped
35 g (1¼ oz/¼ cup) pistachio nuts, chopped
2 tbsp lemon juice
2 small lemons
2 small red onions
olive or canola oil spray

PREP TIME: 20 MINUTES + MARINATING TIME
COOKING TIME: 10 MINUTES
SERVES 4–6

Cut the lamb into 3 cm (1¼ in) cubes. Combine the Moroccan seasoning, lemon juice and garlic in a non-metallic bowl, then add the meat. Cover and refrigerate for 20 minutes.

To make the raita, combine all the ingredients in a bowl. Set aside.

Put the bulgur in a bowl and cover with warm water. Stand for 20 minutes. Drain and squeeze out excess water using clean hands. Return bulgur to bowl and stir through the tomatoes, parsley, mint, dried fruit and nuts. Drizzle with lemon juice. Set aside.

Preheat the oven grill (broiler) or barbecue grill. Cut each lemon into 8 wedges. Cut each onion into 8 wedges. Thread the lamb, lemon and onion wedges alternately onto 8 x 30 cm (12 in) metal skewers. Spray with the oil and brush with any remaining marinade. Grill (broil) and turn for 10 minutes, or until the meat is cooked to your liking.

Serve the kebabs on a bed of bulgur salad and accompany with the raita.

nutrition per serve: Energy 3201 kJ (765 Cal); Fat 13.6 g; Saturated fat 3.9 g; Protein 59.4 g; Carbohydrate 85 g; Fibre 22.9; Cholesterol 127 mg

MONGOLIAN HOTPOT

HOTPOTS ARE A GREAT WAY TO INCLUDE A VARIETY OF HEALTHY FOODS
IN ONE MEAL. THIS SPICY DISH IS A GOOD SOURCE OF IRON, ZINC AND
B-GROUP VITAMINS AND PROVIDES A SATISFYING LOW-GI MEAL.

400 g (14 oz) fresh rice noodles

600 g (1 lb 5 oz) lean lamb backstraps or
   loin fillet

4 spring onions (scallions), sliced

1.5 litres (52 fl oz/6 cups) reduced-salt
   chicken stock

6 thin slices ginger

2 tbsp Chinese rice wine (optional)

300 g (10½ oz) silken firm tofu, cut into
   1.5 cm (⅝ in) cubes

300 g (10½ oz) Chinese broccoli (gai larn),
   cut into 4 cm (1½ in) lengths

150 g (5½ oz/3 cups) shredded Chinese
   cabbage

SAUCE

4 tbsp reduced-sodium soy sauce

2 tbsp Chinese sesame paste

1 tbsp Chinese rice wine (optional)

1 tsp chilli and garlic paste

PREP TIME: 20 MINUTES

COOKING TIME: 5 MINUTES

SERVES 6

Put the noodles in a large heatproof bowl. Cover with boiling water and soak for
8 minutes, or until softened. Separate gently and drain. Divide among 6 bowls.

Trim the lamb, then thinly slice across the grain. Divide the lamb strips among the bowls,
then add spring onion.

Pour the stock into a 2.5 litre (87 fl oz/10 cup) flameproof hotpot or large saucepan, then
add the ginger and rice wine (if using). Cover and bring to the boil over high heat. Add the
tofu, Chinese broccoli and Chinese cabbage and simmer, uncovered, for 1 minute, or until
the broccoli has wilted.

To make the sauce, combine the soy sauce, sesame paste, rice wine and chilli and garlic
paste in a small bowl.

Divide the tofu, broccoli and cabbage among the bowls, then ladle on the hot stock—it will
be hot enough to cook the lamb. Drizzle a little of the sauce on top and serve the rest on
the side.

nutrition per serve: Energy 1665 kJ (396 Cal); Fat 12.7 g; Saturated fat 3.1 g; Protein 35.8 g;
Carbohydrate 32.6 g; Fibre 5.3 g; Cholesterol 65 mg

TUNA WITH LIME AND CHILLI SAUCE AND GREEN VEGETABLES

SAUCE
2 large handfuls mint, chopped
2 large handfuls coriander (cilantro) leaves, chopped
1 tsp grated lime zest
1 tbsp lime juice
1 tsp grated fresh ginger
1 jalapeño chilli, seeded and finely chopped
250 g (9 oz/1 cup) low-fat plain yoghurt

olive canola oil spray
4 tuna steaks
175 g (6 oz) asparagus, trimmed and cut into 5 cm (2 in) pieces
125 g (4½ oz) snow peas (mangetout), trimmed
125 g (4½ oz) green beans, trimmed
4 wholegrain bread rolls, to serve

PREP TIME: 20 MINUTES
COOKING TIME: 10 MINUTES
SERVES 4

To make the sauce, combine the mint, coriander, lime zest, lime juice, ginger and chilli. Fold in the yoghurt and season with freshly ground black pepper.

Heat a chargrill pan over high heat and lightly spray with the oil. Cook the tuna steaks for 2 minutes on each side, or until cooked, but still pink in the centre.

Meanwhile, steam the vegetables for 2–3 minutes, or until just tender.

Top the tuna with the sauce. Serve with the vegetables and bread rolls.

HINT:
• Jalapeño chillies are smooth and thick-fleshed and are available both red and green. They are quite fiery, so you can use a less powerful variety of chilli if you prefer.

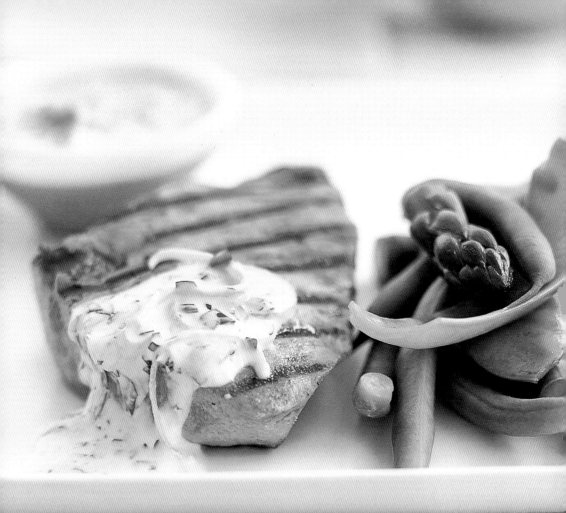

THIS DELICIOUS MEAL IS
QUICK AND EASY TO MAKE AND
PROVIDES USEFUL AMOUNTS OF
NUTRIENTS THAT MANY PEOPLE
DON'T EAT ENOUGH OF—
OMEGA-3 FATTY ACIDS, IRON,
ZINC AND OTHER MINERALS.

nutrition per serve: Energy 1927 kJ (460 Cal)
Fat 12.3 g
Saturated fat 4 g
Protein 51.1 g
Carbohydrate 32.1 g
Fibre 5.6 g
Cholesterol 61 mg

GREEN LENTIL AND VEGETABLE CURRY

IF YOU LIKE A LITTLE SPICE IN YOUR MEALS THIS ONE'S PERFECT. IT'S LOW GI, RICH IN FIBRE AND ALSO CONTAINS A RANGE OF HEALTHY PLANT FOOD COMPOUNDS.

1 tsp olive or canola oil
1 large onion, chopped
2 garlic cloves, chopped
1–2 tbsp curry paste
1 tsp ground turmeric
200 g (7 oz/1 cup) green lentils, rinsed and drained
1.25 litres (44 fl oz/5 cups) reduced-salt vegetable stock
1 large carrot, cut into 2 cm (¾ in) cubes
375 g (13 oz) sweet potato, peeled and cut into 2 cm (¾ in) cubes

2 zucchini (courgettes), cut into 2 cm (¾ in) slices
2 baby eggplant (aubergine), cut into 1 cm (½ in) slices
basmati or wild rice, to serve (see Hint)
basil, to serve
coriander (cilantro) leaves, to serve

PREP TIME: 20 MINUTES
COOKING TIME: 1 HOUR 5 MINUTES
SERVES 4

Heat the oil in a saucepan over a medium heat. Add the onion and garlic and cook for 3 minutes, or until softened. Stir in the curry paste and turmeric and stir for 1 minute. Add the lentils and stock or water.

Bring to the boil, then reduce the heat. Cover and simmer for 30 minutes, then add the carrot and sweet potato. Simmer, covered, for 20 minutes, or until the lentils and vegetables are tender.

Add the zucchini and eggplant, cover and simmer for 10 minutes, or until the vegetables are cooked and most of the liquid has been absorbed. Remove the lid and simmer for a further few minutes if there is too much liquid. Serve hot with basmati rice or wild rice and top with basil and coriander leaves.

HINT:
• The rice will add a lot more carbohydrate, so if you have difficulty controlling your blood sugar level make sure that you have no more than 1 cup of cooked rice.

nutrition per serve: Energy 1321 kJ (316 Cal); Fat 6.2 g; Saturated fat 0.8 g; Protein 16.9 g; Carbohydrate 43.2 g; Fibre 15.2 g; Cholesterol 0 mg

CORIANDER BEEF WITH NOODLES

Marinate the beef overnight or during the day to allow the flavours to develop in this tasty dish. The lime juice and coriander give a tangy flavour boost.

MARINADE
4 garlic cloves, finely chopped
1 tbsp finely chopped fresh ginger
1 large handful coriander (cilantro) roots, stems and leaves, chopped
3 tsp olive or canola oil

500 g (1 lb 2 oz) lean beef rump steak
400 g (14 oz) fresh rice noodles
olive or canola oil spray
1 red onion, thinly sliced

½ red capsicum (pepper), thinly sliced
½ green capsicum (pepper), thinly sliced
2 tbsp lime juice
2 tbsp reduced-sodium soy sauce
1 large handful coriander (cilantro) leaves, extra

Prep time: 20 minutes + 2 hours marinating
Cooking time: 20 minutes
Serves 4

To make the marinade, combine the garlic, ginger, coriander and 2 teaspoons of the oil in a large non-metallic bowl. Trim the beef, then cut into thin strips across the grain. Add to the marinade and toss to coat. Cover with plastic wrap and refrigerate for 2 hours, or overnight.

Put the rice noodles in a large heatproof bowl, cover with boiling water and soak for 8 minutes, or until softened. Separate gently and drain.

Heat a wok until very hot over high heat and spray with the oil. Add the meat in three batches and stir-fry for 2–3 minutes, or until the meat is just cooked. Remove all the meat from the wok and keep it warm. Reheat and respray the wok between batches.

Heat the remaining 1 teaspoon of oil in the wok. Add the onion and cook over medium heat for 3–4 minutes, or until slightly softened. Add the capsicum and cook, tossing constantly, for 3–4 minutes, or until slightly softened.

Return all the meat to the wok along with the lime juice, soy sauce, 2 tablespoons of water and extra coriander. Add the noodles. Toss well, then remove from the heat and season well with freshly ground black pepper.

nutrition per serve: Energy 1712 kJ (409 Cal); Fat 10.4 g; Saturated fat 2.8 g; Protein 32.6 g; Carbohydrate 43.9 g; Fibre 2.2 g; Cholesterol 80 mg

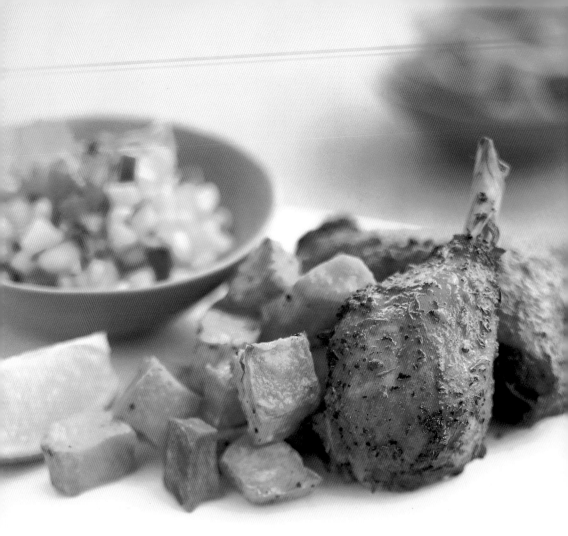

THIS LOWER FAT, HEALTHIER VERSION OF CHICKEN AND CHIPS IS RICH WITH EXOTIC FLAVOURS. THE DIFFERENT VEGETABLES GIVE YOU A RANGE OF ANTIOXIDANTS AND PHYTOCHEMICALS.

nutrition per serve: Energy 2013 kJ (481 Cal)
Fat 13.6 g
Saturated fat 3.7 g
Protein 41 g
Carbohydrate 44.4 g
Fibre 7.2 g
Cholesterol 155 mg

CAJUN CHICKEN WITH SALSA

4 sweet potatoes, peeled and cut into
   3 cm (1¼ in) chunks
olive or canola oil spray
4 skinless chicken thighs on the bone
4 skinless chicken drumsticks
3 tbsp Cajun seasoning
lime wedges, to serve

SALSA
3 cobs sweet corn
1 Lebanese (short) cucumber, cut into
   5 mm (¼ in) dice

2 vine-ripened tomatoes, cut into 5 mm
   (¼ in) dice
1 small handful coriander (cilantro) leaves,
   roughly chopped
2 tbsp lime juice
1 tsp fish sauce

PREP TIME: 25 MINUTES
COOKING TIME: 50 MINUTES
SERVES 4

Preheat the oven to 180°C (350°F/Gas 4). Spray the sweet potatoes with the oil and season. Place in a roasting tin and roast in the oven for 40–45 minutes, or until golden and cooked through.

Put the chicken in a large bowl, add the Cajun seasoning mix and toss together well until the pieces are evenly coated. Place into a roasting tin and roast in the oven for 45 minutes, or until cooked through.

To make the salsa, cook the corn in a saucepan of boiling water for 8 minutes. Drain and refresh under cold water. Remove the kernels, using a sharp knife, and place in a bowl with the cucumber, tomato, coriander, lime juice and fish sauce. Mix together and season with pepper.

Serve the chicken pieces with the roasted sweet potato, the salsa and lime wedges.

123

PRAWN JAMBALAYA

JAMBALAYA IS A VERSATILE CREOLE DISH THAT COMBINES COOKED RICE WITH
A VARIETY OF VEGETABLES PLUS ANY KIND OF MEAT, POULTRY OR SEAFOOD.
THIS PRAWN-BASED VERSION IS LOW IN FAT AND PROVIDES GOOD AMOUNTS
OF IODINE, SELENIUM AND ZINC.

1 kg (2 lb 4 oz) large prawns (shrimp),
   peeled and deveined, heads, shells and
   tails reserved
2 small onions, chopped
2 sticks celery, chopped
250 ml (9 fl oz/1 cup) reduced-salt chicken
   stock
1 tbsp olive or canola oil
125 g (4½ oz) low-fat bacon (we used 97%
   fat-free), thinly sliced
1 red capsicum (pepper), chopped

400 g (14 oz) tinned chopped tomatoes
½ tsp cayenne pepper
½ tsp black pepper
¼ tsp dried thyme
¼ tsp dried oregano
400 g (14 oz/2 cups) basmati or doongara
   rice

PREP TIME: 25 MINUTES
COOKING TIME: 1 HOUR 10 MINUTES
SERVES 4–6

Put the prawn heads, shells and tails in a saucepan with half the onion, half the celery, the
stock and 1 litre (35 fl oz/4 cups) of water. Bring to the boil, then reduce the heat and
simmer for 20 minutes. Strain through a fine sieve, reserving the prawn stock.

Heat the oil in a large, heavy-based saucepan and cook the bacon for 3 minutes, or until
lightly browned. Remove from the saucepan with a slotted spoon and set aside.

Add the remaining onion, the remaining celery and the capsicum to the saucepan
and cook, stirring occasionally, for 5 minutes. Add the tomato, cayenne pepper, black
pepper and dried herbs and bring to the boil. Reduce the heat and simmer, covered,
for 10 minutes.

Return the bacon to the pan and add the rice and prawn stock. Bring back to the boil,
reduce the heat and simmer, covered, for 25 minutes, or until most of the liquid has been
absorbed and the rice is tender.

Add the prawns to the saucepan and stir through gently. Cover and cook for a further
5 minutes, or until the prawns are pink and cooked through. Serve immediately.

nutrition per serve (6): Energy 1676 kJ (400 Cal); Fat 4.8 g; Saturated fat 0.7 g; Protein 29.5 g;
Carbohydrate 58.3 g; Fibre 2.3 g; Cholesterol 144 mg

CHILLI CON CARNE

THIS SPICY CLASSIC PROVIDES A SUSTAINING LOW-GI MEAL WITH SIGNIFICANT AMOUNTS OF VITAMIN C, FOLATE, BETACAROTENE, B-GROUP VITAMINS, IRON AND ZINC.

2 tsp olive or canola oil
1 large onion, chopped
1 garlic clove, crushed
1 tsp cayenne pepper
2 tsp paprika
1 tsp dried oregano
2 tsp ground cumin
750 g (1 lb 10 oz) extra lean minced (ground) beef
375 ml (13 lf oz/1½ cups) reduced-salt beef stock
400 g (14 oz) tinned diced tomatoes

125 g (4½ oz/½ cup) no-added-salt tomato paste (concentrated purée)
300 g (10½ oz) tinned kidney beans, drained and rinsed
fresh flat-leaf (Italian) parsley sprigs, to garnish
basmati or doongar rice, to serve (see Hint)

PREP TIME: 15 MINUTES
COOKING TIME: 1 HOUR 10 MINUTES
SERVES 6

Heat the oil in a saucepan over low heat. Add the onion and cook for 4–5 minutes, or until soft. Stir in the garlic, cayenne pepper, paprika, oregano and cumin. Increase the heat to medium, add the minced beef and cook for 5–8 minutes, or until just browned.

Reduce the heat to low and add the stock, tomato and tomato paste. Cook for 40 minutes, stirring frequently.

Stir in the kidney beans and simmer for 10 minutes. Serve the chilli con carne on its own in small bowls or over steamed basmati or doongara rice. Garnish with a sprig of parsley.

HINT:
• The rice will add more carbohydrate, so choose a small serve.

nutrition per serve: Energy 1154 kJ (276 Cal); Fat 10.4 g; Saturated fat 3.9 g; Protein 30.3 g; Carbohydrate 11.7 g; Fibre 4.7 g; Cholesterol 65 mg

REDUCED-FAT LASAGNE

2 tsp olive or canola oil
1 large onion, chopped
2 carrots, finely chopped
2 celery stalks, finely chopped
2 zucchini (courgettes), finely chopped
2 garlic cloves, crushed
500 g (1 lb 2 oz) lean minced (ground) beef
800 g (1 lb 12 oz) tinned chopped
   tomatoes
125 ml (4 fl oz/½ cup) reduced-salt beef
   stock
2 tbsp no-added-salt tomato paste
   (concentrated purée)

2 tsp dried oregano
375 g (13 oz) instant lasagne sheets
mixed-leaf salad with balsamic vinegar,
   to serve

CHEESE SAUCE
750 ml (26 fl oz/3 cups) skim milk
40 g (1½ oz/⅓ cup) cornflour (cornstarch)
100 g (3½ oz) reduced-fat cheddar cheese

PREP TIME: 40 MINUTES
COOKING TIME: 1 HOUR 35 MINUTES
SERVES 8

Heat the oil in a large non-stick saucepan over medium heat. Add the onion and cook for 5 minutes, or until soft. Add the carrot, celery and zucchini and cook, stirring constantly, for 5 minutes, or until soft. Add the garlic and cook for 1 minute. Increase the heat to high, add the beef and cook, stirring, until well browned. Break up any lumps with a wooden spoon. Add the tomato, stock, tomato paste and oregano to the pan and stir well. Bring to the boil, then reduce the heat and simmer gently, partially covered, for 20 minutes, stirring occasionally to prevent the mixture sticking to the pan.

Preheat the oven to 180°C (350°F/Gas 4). Spread a little of the meat sauce into the base of a 23 x 30 cm (9 x 12 in) ovenproof dish. Arrange a layer of lasagne sheets in the dish, breaking some of the sheets, if necessary, to fit in neatly. Spread half the meat sauce over the top to cover evenly. Cover with another layer of lasagne sheets, a layer of meat sauce, then a final layer of lasagne sheets.

To make the cheese sauce, blend a little of the milk with the cornflour, to form a smooth paste, in a small saucepan. Gradually blend in the remaining milk and stir constantly over low heat until the mixture boils and thickens. Remove from the heat and stir in the cheese until melted.

Spread the sauce evenly over the top of the lasagne. Bake for 1 hour, checking after 25 minutes. If the top is browning too quickly, cover loosely with non-stick baking paper or foil sprayed with oil. Take care when removing the paper or foil that the topping does not lift off. Serve with the mixed-leaf salad.

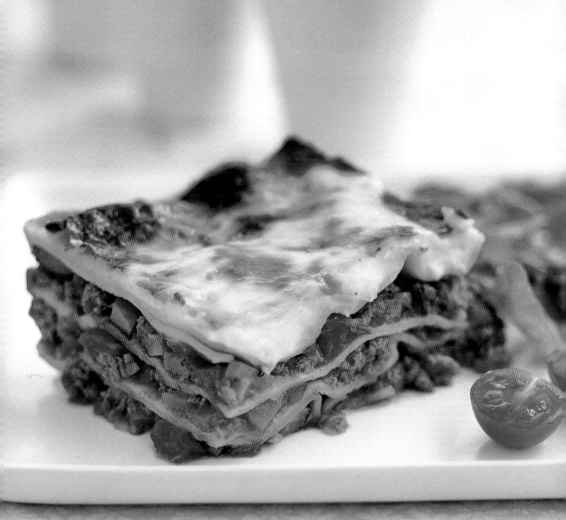

A PERENNIAL FAVOURITE,
THIS VERSION HAS ALL THE
FLAVOUR BUT LESS FAT THAN
TRADITIONAL LASAGNE—BUT
YOU STILL NEED TO LIMIT
YOURSELF TO ONE PORTION.

nutrition per serve: Energy 1393 kJ (333 Cal)
Fat 9 g
Saturated fat 3.8 g
Protein 26.1 g
Carbohydrate 35.3 g
Fibre 5 g
Cholesterol 43 mg

SPAGHETTI BOLOGNESE

THIS IS A LOW-GI DISH THE WHOLE FAMILY WILL ENJOY. MEATY SAUCE GOES WELL WITH MOST TYPES OF PASTA, SO YOU CAN SWAP THE SPAGHETTI WITH OTHER TYPES OF PASTA FOR A NEW TWIST.

olive or canola oil spray
2 onions, finely chopped
2 garlic cloves, finely chopped
2 carrots, finely chopped
2 celery stalks, finely chopped
400 g (14 oz) lean minced (ground) beef
1 kg (2 lb 4 oz) tomatoes, chopped
125 ml (4 fl oz/½ cup) red wine (see Hints)
350 g (12 oz) spaghetti

3 tbsp finely chopped flat-leaf (Italian) parsley
mixed-leaf salad with balsamic vinegar, to serve

PREP TIME: 20 MINUTES

COOKING TIME: 1 HOUR 20 MINUTES

SERVES 6

Heat a large saucepan over medium heat. Spray with the oil, then add the onion, garlic, carrot and celery. Stir for 5 minutes, or until the vegetables have softened. Add 1 tablespoon water, if necessary, to prevent sticking.

Increase the heat to high, add the beef and cook for 5 minutes, or until browned. Stir constantly to prevent the meat sticking. Add the tomatoes, wine and 250 ml (9 fl oz/1 cup) water. Bring to the boil, reduce the heat and simmer, uncovered, for about 1 hour, until the sauce has thickened.

Meanwhile, cook the spaghetti in a large saucepan of boiling water for 10 minutes, or until *al dente*. Drain. Stir the parsley through the sauce, season with salt and freshly ground black pepper and serve over the pasta. Serve with the mixed-leaf salad.

HINTS:
• This dish tastes even better the next day and can be kept in the fridge for up to 2 days or frozen for up to 1 month.
• If you'd prefer not to use wine, the same amount of liquid can be replaced with reduced-salt beef stock.
• Choose wholemeal pasta if you're watching your weight to make this meal more filling.

nutrition per serve: Energy 1495 kJ (357 Cal); Fat 5.9 g; Saturated fat 2.1 g; Protein 22.6 g; Carbohydrate 46.3 g; Fibre 5.5 g; Cholesterol 34 mg

MOUSSAKA

THIS LOW-FAT VERSION OF A GREEK FAVOURITE MAKES A NOURISHING, LOW-GI MEAL, PROVIDING GOOD AMOUNTS OF IRON, ZINC, CALCIUM, PHOSPHORUS, PROTEIN AND VARIOUS ANTIOXIDANTS.

1 kg (2 lb 4 oz) eggplant (aubergine)
olive or canola oil spray
2 onions, finely chopped
3 large garlic cloves, crushed
½ tsp ground allspice
1 tsp ground cinnamon
500 g (1 lb 2 oz) lean minced (ground) lamb
2 tbsp no-added-salt tomato paste
   (concentrated purée)
125 ml (4 fl oz/½ cup) reduced-salt
   vegetable or beef stock
800 g (1 lb 12 oz) tinned tomatoes
3 tbsp chopped flat-leaf (Italian) parsley

90 g (3¼ oz) low-fat cheddar cheese,
   grated
1 tbsp reduced-fat olive oil or canola oil
   margarine
40 g (1½ oz/⅓ cup) plain (all-purpose)
   flour
375 ml (13 fl oz/1½ cups) skim milk
150 g (5½ oz/⅔ cup) low-fat ricotta cheese
pinch ground nutmeg

PREP TIME: 30 MINUTES

COOKING TIME: 1 HOUR 30 MINUTES

SERVES 6

Preheat the oven to 180°C (350°F/Gas 4). Cut the eggplant into 5 mm (¼ in) thick slices. Spray the eggplant with the oil and grill (broil) under a preheated grill (broiler) for 4 minutes on each side, or until golden.

Heat a non-stick saucepan and lightly spray with oil. Cook the onions for 3–4 minutes, or until softened. Add the garlic, allspice and cinnamon and cook for 1 minute. Add the lamb and cook for 3–4 minutes, or until cooked. Add the tomato paste, stock and tomatoes. Bring to the boil, then reduce the heat and simmer for 30–35 minutes, stirring occasionally, or until most of the liquid has evaporated. Stir in the parsley and season.

To make the white sauce, melt the margarine in a saucepan over medium heat. Stir in the flour and cook for 1 minute. Remove from the heat and gradually stir in the milk. Return to the heat and stir constantly until the sauce boils and thickens. Reduce the heat and simmer for 2 minutes. Stir through the ricotta and nutmeg until smooth and season with freshly ground black pepper.

Spoon half the meat sauce into a 3-litre (105 fl oz/12 cup) ovenproof dish. Cover with half of the eggplant. Spoon over the remaining meat sauce and cover with the remaining eggplant. Spread over the sauce and sprinkle with the cheese. Bake for 30 minutes, or until golden.

nutrition per serve: Energy 1409 kJ (337 Cal); Fat 12.5 g; Saturated fat 4.5 g; Protein 31.4 g; Carbohydrate 21.1 g; Fibre 7.3; Cholesterol 66 mg

THIS IS A GOOD WEEKDAY RECIPE
BECAUSE IT DOESN'T TAKE LONG TO
PREPARE. IT'S LOW GI AND A GOOD
SOURCE OF FIBRE, FOLATE,
BETACAROTENE AND LYCOPENE.

nutrition per serve: Energy 2114 kJ (505 Cal)

Fat 4.4 g

Saturated fat 0.6 g

Protein 16.6 g

Carbohydrate 94.5 g

Fibre 7.2 g

Cholesterol 2 mg

PASTA PUTTANESCA

2 tsp olive or canola oil
3 garlic cloves, crushed
2 tbsp chopped flat-leaf (Italian) parsley
$\frac{1}{4}$–$\frac{1}{2}$ tsp chilli flakes or powder
800 g (1 lb 12 oz) tinned chopped
   tomatoes
500 g (1 lb 2 oz) spaghetti
1 tbsp capers
3 anchovy fillets in brine, drained and
   thinly sliced

40 g (1$\frac{1}{2}$ oz/$\frac{1}{4}$ cup) black olives in brine,
   drained, pitted and chopped
mixed-leaf salad with balsamic vinegar,
   to serve

PREP TIME: 20 MINUTES
COOKING TIME: 25 MINUTES
SERVES 4

Heat the oil in a large heavy-based frying pan. Add the garlic, parsley and chilli flakes and stir constantly for about 1 minute over medium heat. Add the tomato to the pan and bring to the boil. Reduce the heat and simmer, covered, for 10 minutes.

Meanwhile, cook the pasta in a large saucepan of boiling water for 10 minutes, or until *al dente*. Drain and return to the pan.

Add the capers, anchovies and olives to the tomato mixture and stir for a further 5 minutes. Season with freshly ground black pepper. Add the sauce to the pasta and toss gently. Serve with the mixed-leaf salad.

HINTS:
• You can substitute the anchovies with a small–medium tin of tuna if you don't like anchovies.
• Less active people need to make sure that they don't overdo the pasta—so eat less pasta and more sauce and salad for a more filling meal.

PENNE WITH SEARED TUNA AND ZUCCHINI

THIS LOW-FAT MEDITERRANEAN-STYLE DISH WITH A HINT OF ZESTY LEMON PROVIDES PLENTY OF PROTEIN, OMEGA-3 FATTY ACIDS, NIACIN, POTASSIUM, FOLATE, AND SOME IRON AND ZINC.

400 g (14 oz) penne pasta
olive or canola oil spray
500 g (1 lb 2 oz) tuna steaks
1 large red onion, cut into thin wedges
2 zucchini (courgettes), sliced into 7 cm
   (2¾ in) long thin strips
1 garlic clove, chopped
6 small gherkins, rinsed and chopped

1 large handful flat-leaf (Italian) parsley,
   chopped
zest and juice from 1 large lemon
mixed-leaf salad with balsamic vinegar,
   to serve

PREP TIME: 15 MINUTES
COOKING TIME: 20 MINUTES
SERVES 4

Cook the pasta in a large saucepan of boiling salted water for 10 minutes, or until *al dente*. Drain, reserving 250 ml (9 fl oz/1 cup) of the pasta water. Return the pasta to the saucepan.

Meanwhile, pat the fish dry with paper towels. Lightly spray a large, non-stick frying pan with the oil. Heat the oil, add the fish and cook for 2–3 minutes on each side, or until browned on the outside and still pink in the centre. Remove the fish from the pan. Set aside for a few minutes, then cut into 2 cm (¾ in) cubes.

Spray the frying pan with more oil and heat the pan. Add the onion, zucchini and garlic and cook for 2–3 minutes, or until softened. Stir in the gherkins, parsley, lemon zest and juice. Toss into the hot pasta together with the fish and enough of the reserved pasta water to moisten. Season with freshly ground black pepper. Serve with the mixed-leaf salad.

HINT:
• If you generally have trouble keeping your blood sugar level under control, make sure you have a smaller serve of pasta. If you feel like seconds, fill up on salad.

nutrition per serve: Energy 2511 kJ (600 Cal); Fat 9.5 g; Saturated fat 3.2 g; Protein 44.2 g; Carbohydrate 79.4 g; Fibre 6.1 g; Cholesterol 45 mg

LENTIL AND RICOTTA LASAGNE

THIS DISH IS LOWER IN FAT THAN REGULAR LASAGNE AND CONTAINS MORE FIBRE. IT IS ALSO LOW IN SATURATED FAT.

90 g (3¼ oz/½ cup) red lentils
1 large onion
1 small red capsicum (pepper)
2 zucchini (courgettes)
1 celery stalk
2 tsp olive or canola oil
2–3 garlic cloves, crushed
800 g (1 lb 12 oz) tinned chopped tomatoes
2 tbsp no-added-salt tomato paste (concentrated purée)
1 tsp dried oregano
40 g (1½ oz/⅓ cup) cornflour (cornstarch)

750 ml (26 fl oz/3 cups) skim milk
¼ onion
½ tsp ground nutmeg
350 g (12 oz/1⅓ cups) low-fat ricotta cheese
12 dried or fresh lasagne sheets
60 g (2¼ oz/½ cup) grated reduced-fat cheddar cheese

PREP TIME: 30 MINUTES + 30 MINUTES SOAKING
COOKING TIME: 1 HOUR 50 MINUTES
SERVES 6

Pour the lentils into a bowl, cover with boiling water and leave to soak for 30 minutes. Drain. Chop the onion and capsicum, then slice the zucchini and celery. Heat the oil in a saucepan, add the garlic and onion and cook for 2 minutes. Add the capsicum, zucchini and celery and cook for 2–3 minutes, or until softened. Add the lentils, tomatoes, tomato paste, oregano and 375 ml (13 fl oz/1½ cups) water. Bring to the boil, then reduce the heat and simmer for 30 minutes, or until the lentils are tender. Preheat the oven to 180°C (350°F/Gas 4).

Blend the cornflour with 2 tablespoons of the milk in a saucepan until smooth. Pour the remaining milk into the pan. Add the onion and stir over low heat until the mixture boils and thickens. Add the nutmeg and season with freshly ground black pepper, then cook over low heat for 5 minutes. Remove the onion.

Beat the ricotta with 125 ml (4 fl oz/½ cup) of the white sauce. Spread one-third of the lentil mixture over the base of a 3 litre (105 fl oz/12 cup) ovenproof dish. Cover with a layer of lasagne sheets. Spread another third of the lentil mixture over the pasta, then spread the ricotta over the top. Follow with another layer of lasagne, then the remaining lentils.

Pour the white sauce over the top. Sprinkle with the grated cheese. Bake for 1 hour, covering with lightly oiled foil if the top starts to brown too much. Stand for 5 minutes before cutting.

nutrition per serve: Energy 1660 kJ (397 Cal); Fat 7.9 g; Saturated fat 2.9 g; Protein 23.7 g; Carbohydrate 55.1 g; Fibre 6.8 g; Cholesterol 10 mg

COQ AU VIN

2 tsp olive or canola oil
125 g (4½ oz) low-fat bacon (we used
 97% fat-free), roughly chopped
1.5 kg (3 lb 5 oz) skinless chicken pieces,
 trimmed
350 g (12 oz) baby onions
2 tbsp plain (all-purpose) flour
750 ml (26 fl oz/3 cups) reduced-salt beef
 stock

250 g (9 oz) field mushrooms, sliced
1 tbsp thyme, to garnish
6 wholegrain bread rolls

PREP TIME: 15 MINUTES
COOKING TIME: 1 HOUR 50 MINUTES
SERVES 6

Preheat the oven to 180°C (350°F/Gas 4). Heat the oil in a large flameproof casserole dish. Add the bacon and cook until golden, then remove. Add the chicken in batches and cook for 4–5 minutes, or until browned. Remove from the dish. Add the onions and cook for 2–3 minutes, or until browned, then remove from the dish.

Add the flour to the dish and stir well, then remove from the heat and slowly stir in the stock. Return to the heat, bring to the boil and return the bacon and chicken to the pan. Cover and cook in the oven for 1 hour. Return the onions to the pan and add the mushrooms. Cook for a further 30 minutes. Season to taste with freshly ground black pepper, then garnish with the thyme.

Meanwhile, put the bread rolls in the oven for a few minutes, or until warmed through. Serve with the casserole.

HINT:
• For extra filling power and antioxidants, serve with a medley of steamed vegetables, such as broccoli, cauliflower, squash, carrots and zucchini (courgette).

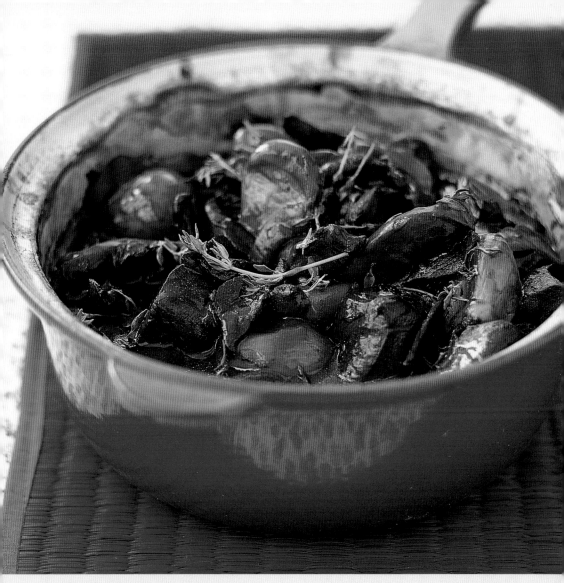

THIS RECIPE CONTAINS LESS
FAT THAN THE TRADITIONAL
FRENCH VERSION OF COQ
AU VIN, BUT STILL HAS ALL
THE FLAVOUR. IT'S GREAT
AS LEFTOVERS.

nutrition per serve: Energy 2158 kJ (515 Cal)

Fat 19.4 g

Saturated fat 5.6 g

Protein 49.2 g

Carbohydrate 34 g

Fibre 5.2 g

Cholesterol 150 mg

OSSO BUCCO WITH GREMOLATA

A GREAT WINTER WARMER, OSSO BUCCO CAN BE SERVED WITH PASTA OR GRAINY BREAD FOR A NOURISHING LOW-GI MEAL.

GREMOLATA
1 tbsp finely shredded lemon zest
1–2 garlic cloves, finely chopped
3 tbsp finely chopped flat-leaf (Italian) parsley

plain (all-purpose) flour, for dusting
4 lean veal shank pieces, 5 cm (2 in) thick
2 tsp olive or canola oil
2 large onions, sliced
6 roma (plum) tomatoes, finely chopped
2 tbsp no-added-salt tomato paste (concentrated purée)

375 ml (13 fl oz/1½ cups) white wine
1 tbsp cornflour (cornstarch)
2–3 garlic cloves, crushed
60 g (2¼ oz) flat-leaf (Italian) parsley, finely chopped
375 g (13 oz) penne
mixed-leaf salad with balsamic vinegar, to serve

PREP TIME: 40 MINUTES
COOKING TIME: 2½ HOURS
SERVES 4

To make the gremolata, mix together the lemon zest, garlic and parsley and set aside.

Season the flour with a little salt and freshly ground black pepper. Toss the veal pieces in the flour, shaking off any excess. Heat half the oil in a large heavy-based frying pan. When the oil is hot, brown the veal on both sides. Remove and set aside.

Heat the remaining oil in the pan and cook the onion for 2–3 minutes, or until soft but not brown. Add the meat in a single layer so that it fits snugly in the pan. Season with freshly ground black pepper.

Mix together the tomatoes, tomato paste and wine and pour the mixture over the meat. Bring to the boil, then reduce the heat, cover and simmer for 1½ hours.

Remove 250 ml (9 fl oz/1 cup) of the cooking liquid and set aside to cool slightly. Put the cornflour in a small bowl and whisk in the reserved liquid, then stir in the garlic and chopped parsley and add the mixture to the pan. Simmer, uncovered, for about 30 minutes, or until the meat is very tender and the sauce has thickened. Sprinkle with the gremolata just before serving.

Meanwhile, cook the pasta in a large saucepan of boiling water for 10 minutes, or until *al dente*. Drain well. Serve with the mixed-leaf salad.

nutrition per serve: Energy 2461 kJ (588 Cal); Fat 6.5 g; Saturated fat 1.3 g; Protein 33.4 g; Carbohydrate 77.1 g; Fibre 7.5 g; Cholesterol 75 mg

CHILLI BEANS WITH POLENTA

SUITABLE FOR VEGETARIANS WHO EAT DAIRY PRODUCTS, THIS DELIGHTFULLY SPICY DISH IS RICH IN FIBRE AND PROVIDES COMPLETE PROTEIN PLUS GOOD AMOUNTS OF FIBRE AND ANTIOXIDANTS.

420 g (14½ oz) tinned creamed corn

375 ml (13 fl oz/1½ cups) reduced-salt
vegetable stock

70 g (2½ oz/½ cup) instant polenta
(see Hint)

310 g (10½ oz) tinned corn kernels, drained

40 g (1½ oz/⅓ cup) low-fat vintage
cheddar cheese, grated

1 tbsp chopped coriander (cilantro) leaves

1 tbsp olive oil

1 red onion, sliced

2 garlic cloves, crushed

1 tsp chilli powder

1 tsp paprika

1 tbsp ground cumin

1 tsp ground coriander

400 g (14 oz) tinned kidney beans, rinsed
and drained

400 g (14 oz) tinned borlotti beans, rinsed
and drained

800 g (1 lb 12 oz) tinned tomatoes

2 tbsp no-added-salt tomato paste
(conentrated pureé)

2 tbsp chopped coriander (cilantro) leaves

PREP TIME: 15 MINUTES

COOKING TIME: 35 MINUTES

SERVES 6

Line a 20 cm (8 in) round cake tin with plastic wrap. Place the creamed corn and stock in a saucepan and bring to the boil. Stir in the polenta and corn kernels, and cook over a medium heat until it comes away from the sides. Stir in the cheese and coriander, cool for 5 minutes, then spoon into the tin and level the surface. Cool.

Heat the oil in a large saucepan, add the onion, garlic and spices and cook until soft. Stir in the beans, tomato and tomato paste. Simmer for 20 minutes. Stir in the coriander.

Lift the polenta from the tin with the aid of the plastic wrap, cut into wedges and serve with the chilli beans and a salad on the side.

HINT:
• The coarser the polenta, the lower the GI (using a thicker polenta rather than very fine instant polenta is recommeneded).

nutrition per serve: Energy 1367 kJ (327 Cal); Fat 5.9 g; Saturated fat 1.1 g; Protein 13.8 g; Carbohydrate 50 g; Fibre 11.2 g; Cholesterol 7 mg

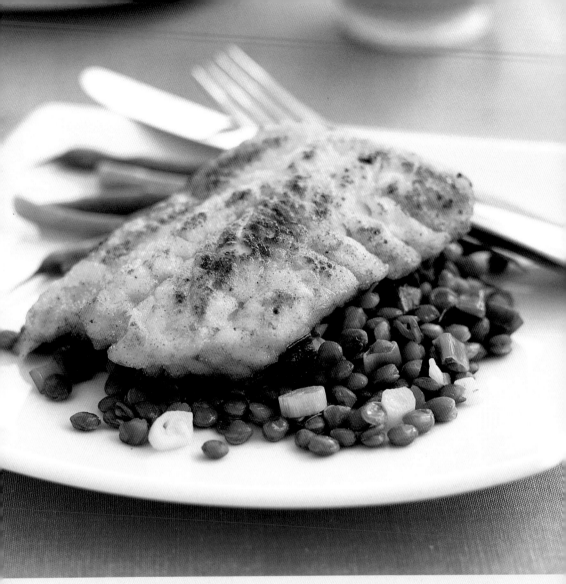

THIS DISH IS HEALTHIER THAN
FISH AND CHIPS WITH MUCH
LESS FAT AND MORE
NUTRIENTS. IT COMBINES THE
FILLING POWERS OF FISH AND
LENTILS TO GIVE YOU A VERY
SATISFYING MEAL.

nutrition per serve: Energy 1416 kJ (338 Cal)
Fat 10.4 g
Saturated fat 0.8 g
Protein 36.6 g
Carbohydrate 21.1 g
Fibre 6 g
Cholesterol 49 mg

CRISPY FISH AND LENTILS

55 g (2 oz/⅓ cup) plain (all-purpose) flour

4 (600 g/1 lb 5 oz) boneless white
   fish fillets

2 tbsp olive or canola oil

4 spring onions (scallions), diagonally
   sliced

2 garlic cloves, crushed

800 g (1 lb 12 oz) tinned brown lentils,
   drained

250 g (9 oz) green beans, trimmed

PREP TIME: 10 MINUTES

COOKING TIME: 15 MINUTES

SERVES 4

Coat the fish fillets in the flour, shaking off any excess. Heat 1 tablespoon of the oil in a large non-stick frying pan over medium–high heat. Add the fish and cook for 3–4 minutes on each side, or until cooked through and lightly browned—depending on the size of your frying pan you may need to cook the fish in batches.

Meanwhile, heat the remaining oil in a large saucepan. Cook the spring onions and garlic for 2 minutes, or until softened. Add the lentils. Toss for a few minutes, or until the lentils are heated through.

Steam or microwave the beans for a few minutes, or until just tender.

Serve the fish with the warm lentils and green beans.

HINT:
• You could serve this dish with extra vegetables, such as mushrooms, broccoli, cauliflower or spinach if you want a more filling meal.

ROAST CHICKEN WITH VEGETABLES

INSTEAD OF THE TRADITIONAL STAPLE OF ROAST MEAT AND THREE VEG, TRY THIS DISH OF CHICKEN WITH FIVE DIFFERENT TYPES OF VEGETABLES. IT HAS MORE NUTRIENTS AND COLOUR.

1.4 kg (3 lb) chicken
1 lemon, halved
6 garlic cloves, unpeeled
6 sprigs thyme
400 g (14 oz) orange sweet potato, cut into
   5 cm (2 in) pieces
2 large carrots, peeled and cut into 5cm
   (2 in) pieces
olive or canola oil spray
2 tbsp plain (all-purpose) flour
1 tbsp Dijon mustard

375 ml (13 fl oz/1½ cups) salt-reduced
   chicken stock
4 corn cobs, trimmed
400 g (14 oz) broccoli, cut into florets
2 zucchini (courgettes), cut into 3 cm
   (1¼ in) pieces

PREP TIME: 30 MINUTES
COOKING TIME: 1 HOUR 10 MINUTES
SERVES 4–6

Preheat the oven to 200°C (400°F/Gas 6). Season the chicken and place the lemon in the cavity. Bend the wings back and tuck behind the body of the chicken. Tie the drumsticks together using string or skewers. Place the chicken in a large roasting tin and arrange the garlic, thyme, sweet potato and carrot around it. Spray the chicken and vegetables with the oil, and bake for 1 hour, or until the chicken is tender and the juices run clear. Turn the vegetables after 30 minutes.

Transfer the chicken and vegetables, except the garlic, to separate plates, cover and keep warm. In a large saucepan of boiling water, cook the corn for 8 minutes. Steam the broccoli and zucchini until just tender.

Meanwhile, pour off any excess fat from the roasting tin. Peel the garlic and mash with a fork in the tin. Heat the tin on the stove top, add the flour and cook over medium heat, stirring, until golden. Remove from the heat and stir in the mustard and stock. Return to the heat and stir until the gravy boils and thickens. Carve the chicken and serve skinless portions of meat with the gravy, roast vegetables, corn, broccoli and zucchini.

HINTS:
• Microwave the corn, beans and zucchini if you prefer.
• Make sure you serve the chicken without the skin—that's where most of the fat is.

nutrition per serve: Energy 2458 kJ (587 Cal); Fat 18 g; Saturated fat 4.7 g; Protein 61.2 g; Carbohydrate 38.8 g; Fibre 11.2 g; Cholesterol 188 mg

PEPPER BEEF ON CANNELLINI BEAN MASH

THIS STEAK RECIPE IS LOW IN FAT, BUT RICH IN FLAVOUR AND IS A GOOD SOURCE OF FIBRE, PROTEIN, IRON AND ZINC.

6 garlic cloves, unpeeled

2 tbsp whole black peppercorns

¼ tsp or less sea salt

4 x 160 g (5½ oz) lean beef fillet steaks, trimmed

olive or canola oil spray

500 g (1 lb 2 oz) broccoli, cut into florets

4 tbsp reduced-salt vegetable stock

800 g (1 lb 12 oz) tinned cannellini beans, rinsed and drained

2 tbsp chopped flat-leaf (Italian) parsley

300 g (10½ oz) baby English spinach leaves, trimmed

PREP TIME: 15 MINUTES

COOKING TIME: 40 MINUTES

SERVES 4

Preheat the oven to 180°C (350°F/Gas 4). Roast the garlic on a tray for 20 minutes, or until softened.

Place the peppercorns in a spice grinder (or use a mortar and pestle) with the sea salt, and roughly crush. Put on a plate, then roll the steaks in the mix until they are well coated.

Over medium heat, heat a chargrill pan, spray with the oil, then add the steaks. Cook for 5 minutes on each side for a medium–rare steak. Remove from the pan and rest, covered, for 2 minutes. Steam or microwave the broccoli for 3 minutes, or until just tender.

Squeeze the garlic from the skin and discard the skin. In a saucepan, bring the vegetable stock to the boil. Add the cannellini beans and garlic and roughly crush together, using a fork, until mashed but still quite chunky. When heated stir through the parsley.

Place the spinach in a saucepan with 2 teaspoons water, cover and place over low–medium heat and cook for 1 minute, or until the leaves are just beginning to wilt. Remove from the heat, stir and season well with freshly ground black pepper.

To serve, divide the bean mash and broccoli between 4 serving plates, top the mash with the spinach and sit the fillet on top. Drizzle with any of the juices which may have come from the resting steaks.

nutrition per serve: Energy 1683 kJ (402 Cal); Fat 9.8 g; Saturated fat 3.6 g; Protein 51.7 g; Carbohydrate 19.5 g; Fibre 16.9 g; Cholesterol 109 mg

SLOW-COOKED LAMB SHANKS WITH BARLEY

2 tsp olive or canola oil
4 lean lamb shanks
2 red onions, sliced
10 garlic cloves, peeled
400 g (14 oz) tinned chopped tomatoes
125 ml (4 fl oz/½ cup) reduced-salt
   vegetable stock or dry white wine
1 bay leaf
1 tsp grated lemon zest

1 large red capsicum (pepper), chopped
325 g (11½ oz/1½ cups) pearl barley
3 tbsp chopped flat-leaf (Italian) parsley
mixed-leaf salad with balsamic vinegar,
   to serve

PREP TIME: 20 MINUTES
COOKING TIME: 3¼ HOURS
SERVES 4

Preheat the oven to 170°C (325°F/Gas 3). Heat the oil in a large flameproof casserole dish, add the shanks in batches and cook over high heat until browned on all sides. Remove the lamb to a side plate.

Add the onion and garlic to the dish and cook until softened. Return all the lamb to the casserole dish. Add the tomato, wine, bay leaf, lemon zest, capsicum and 125 ml (4 fl oz/½ cup) water and bring to the boil. Cover the dish and cook in the oven for 2–2½ hours, or until the meat is tender and falling off the bone and the sauce has thickened.

Meanwhile, wash the barley, then drain well. Put it in a large saucepan with 1.25 litres (44 fl oz/5 cups) water. Bring to the boil, then simmer for 30 minutes, or until soft. Drain.

Season the shanks with freshly ground black pepper to taste. Sprinkle the parsley over the top before serving. Serve with the barley and the salad.

HINT:
• Barley is a good source of soluble fibre and a very low-GI food—great for people with diabetes. It is very filling, so some people might find it difficult to eat at first.

THIS IS A PERFECT COUNTRY-STYLE MEAL FOR COLD WINTER WEEKENDS. THE LOW-GI, FIBRE-RICH BARLEY WILL KEEP YOU FULL FOR HOURS.

nutrition per serve: Energy 2505 kJ (598 Cal)
Fat 17.9 g
Saturated fat 6.6 g
Protein 39.5 g
Carbohydrate 57.8 g
Fibre 13 g
Cholesterol 95 mg

PORK AND BEAN CHILLI

THIS DISH IS AN EASY WAY TO INCLUDE LEGUMES IN YOUR DIET.

olive or canola oil spray
600 g (1 lb 5 oz) lean pork fillet
1 small red onion, finely chopped
3 garlic cloves, finely chopped
1½ tsp ground cumin
1 tsp ground oregano
1–1½ tsp dried chilli powder
2 tsp sweet paprika
1 tbsp red wine vinegar
850 g (1 lb 14 oz) tinned kidney beans, drained and rinsed
425 g (15 oz) tinned Italian tomatoes
375 ml (13 fl oz/1½ cups) reduced-salt beef stock

1 tbsp no-added-salt tomato paste (concentrated pureé)
1 dried bay leaf

CORIANDER RICE
250 g (9 oz/1¼ cups) basmati or doongara rice
2–3 tbsp chopped coriander (cilantro) leaves

PREP TIME: 15 MINUTES +10 MINUTES STANDING
COOKING TIME: 2 HOURS
SERVES 4

Heat a large, non-stick saucepan over high heat. Cut the pork into 2.5 cm (1 in) cubes. Spray with the oil, then brown the pork in 2 batches for 2–3 minutes, or until evenly browned. Remove the pork. Reduce the heat to medium, spray the pan with the oil, then add the onion and cook for 4–5 minutes, or until soft. Stir in the garlic, cumin, oregano, chilli and paprika. Add the vinegar and stir for 30 seconds, or until it evaporates.

Return the pork and any juices to the pan, then add the kidney beans, tomatoes and juice, stock, tomato paste and bay leaf. Stir to combine thoroughly and allow the mixture to come to the boil. Reduce the heat to very low and cook, covered, for 1 hour, stirring frequently. Remove the lid from the pan and continue to cook, uncovered, for a further 30 minutes, or until the meat is tender and the sauce has reduced and thickened.

Rinse the rice and put it in a saucepan. Add 425 ml (15 fl oz/1¾ cups) water and bring to the boil. Cover, reduce the heat to low and cook for 10 minutes. Remove from the heat and leave to stand, covered, for 10 minutes.

Season the pork and bean chilli with freshly ground black pepper. Stir the coriander through the rice. Place the rice into 4 serving bowls, top with the pork and bean chilli. Garnish with 2 tablespoons chopped flat-leaf (Italian) parsley, 1 tablespoon chopped coriander and 2 teaspoons extra-light sour cream or low-fat yogurt per serve, if you like.

nutrition per serve: Energy 2429 kJ (580 Cal); Fat 6.1 g; Saturated fat 1.6 g; Protein 48.8 g; Carbohydrate 75.1 g; Fibre 11.9 g; Cholesterol 144 mg

VEAL CUTLETS IN CHILLI TOMATO SAUCE

SERVED WITH A SPICY TOMATO SAUCE, THIS LOW-GI VEAL DISH IS A PERFECT CHOICE FOR WINTER NIGHTS. IT'S A GOOD SOURCE OF PROTEIN, B VITAMINS, FOLATE, POTASSIUM, IRON AND ZINC.

5 slices wholegrain bread

3 tbsp flat-leaf (Italian) parsley

3 garlic cloves

4 thick veal cutlets, trimmed

3 tbsp skim milk

2 tsp olive or canola oil

1 onion, finely chopped

1 tbsp capers, drained

1 tsp canned green peppercorns, chopped

1 tsp chopped red chilli

2 tbsp balsamic vinegar

1 tsp soft brown sugar

2 tbsp no-added-salt tomato paste (concentrated purée)

440 g (15½ oz) tinned chopped tomatoes

PREP TIME: 35 MINUTES

COOKING TIME: 35 MINUTES

SERVES 4

Preheat the oven to 180°C (350°F/Gas 4). Place a rack in a small baking dish. Chop the bread, parsley and garlic in a food processor to make fine breadcrumbs.

Season the cutlets on both sides with a little salt and freshly ground black pepper. Pour the milk into a bowl and put the breadcrumbs on a plate. Dip the veal in the milk, then coat in the crumbs, pressing the crumbs on. Transfer to the rack and bake for 20 minutes.

Meanwhile, heat the oil in a small pan over medium heat. Add the onion, capers, peppercorns and chilli, cover and cook for 8 minutes. Stir in the vinegar, sugar and tomato paste, and stir until boiling. Stir in the tomato, reduce the heat and simmer for 15 minutes, then season with pepper.

Remove the cutlets from the rack and wipe the dish. Place about three-quarters of the tomato sauce in the base and put the cutlets on top. Spoon the remaining sauce over the cutlets and return to the oven. Reduce the oven to 150°C (300°F/Gas 2), then bake for another 10 minutes, or until heated through. Sprinkle with extra chopped parsley.

nutrition per serve: Energy 1316 kJ (314 Cal); Fat 6.9 g; Saturated fat 1.4 g; Protein 33.2 g; Carbohydrate 26.4 g; Fibre 4.9 g; Cholesterol 103 mg

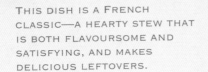

THIS DISH IS A FRENCH
CLASSIC—A HEARTY STEW THAT
IS BOTH FLAVOURSOME AND
SATISFYING, AND MAKES
DELICIOUS LEFTOVERS.

nutrition per serve: Energy 2192 kJ (524 Cal)

Fat 9.7 g

Saturated fat 3.6 g

Protein 48.8 g

Carbohydrate 51.1 g

Fibre 3.4 g

Cholesterol 110 mg

BEEF BOURGUIGNON

1 kg (2 lb 4 oz) lean topside or round steak
plain (all-purpose) flour, for dusting
50 g (1¾ oz) low-fat bacon slices (we used
  97% fat-free)
2 tsp olive or canola oil
12 baby onions
250 ml (9 fl oz/1 cup) red wine (see Hints)
500 ml (17 fl oz/2 cups) reduced-salt beef
  stock
1 tsp dried thyme

200 g (7 oz) button mushrooms
2 bay leaves
375 g (13 oz) fettucine
mixed-leaf salad with balsamic vinegar,
  to serve

PREP TIME: 20 MINUTES
COOKING TIME: 2 HOURS
SERVES 6

Trim the steak and cut into 2 cm (¾ in) cubes. Season the flour with a little salt and freshly ground black pepper. Lightly toss the steak in the flour, shaking off the excess.

Cut the bacon into 2 cm (¾ in) squares. Heat the oil in a large heavy-based saucepan and briefly cook the bacon over medium heat. Remove the bacon from the pan, then add the meat and brown well in batches. Remove and set aside. Add the onions to the pan and cook until golden.

Return the bacon and meat to the pan with the remaining ingredients (except the pasta and salad). Bring to the boil, reduce the heat and simmer, covered, for 1½ hours, or until the meat is very tender, stirring occasionally. Remove the bay leaves to serve.

Meanwhile, cook the pasta in a large saucepan of boiling water for 10 minutes, or until *al dente*. Drain well. Serve with the beef. Serve with the mixed-leaf salad.

HINTS:
• If you'd prefer not to use wine, the same amount of liquid can be replaced with extra reduced-salt beef stock.
• Great as leftovers, this dish will keep refrigerated in an airtight container for up to 3 days.

CHICKEN CHASSEUR

THIS NOURISHING STEW IS PERFECT IN COOL WEATHER. MAKE IT ON THE WEEKEND WHEN YOU HAVE PLENTY OF TIME TO ENJOY THE SUCCULENT AROMAS WHILE IT'S COOKING.

2 tsp olive or canola oil
1 kg (2 lb 4 oz) skinless chicken thigh
  fillets, trimmed
1 garlic clove, crushed
1 large onion, sliced
100 g (3½ oz) button mushrooms, sliced
1 tsp thyme
400 g (14 oz) tinned tomatoes
3 tbs reduced-salt chicken stock

3 tbsp white wine (optional)
1 tbsp no-added-salt tomato paste
  (concentrated purée)
375 g (13 oz) penne

PREP TIME: 20 MINUTES

COOKING TIME: 1 HOUR 30 MINUTES

SERVES 4

Preheat the oven to 180°C (350°F/Gas 4). Heat the oil in a heavy-based frying pan and brown the chicken in batches over medium heat. Drain on paper towels, then transfer to a casserole dish.

Add the garlic, onion and mushrooms to the pan and cook over medium heat for 5 minutes, or until soft. Add to the chicken with the thyme and tomatoes and crush the tomatoes with a wooden spoon. Season with freshly ground black pepper.

Combine the stock, wine and tomato paste and pour over the chicken. Cover and bake for 1¼ hours, or until the chicken is tender.

Meanwhile, cook the pasta in a large saucepan of boiling water for 10 minutes, or until *al dente*. Drain well. Serve with the chicken.

nutrition per serve: Energy 3066 kJ (730 Cal); Fat 21.7 g; Saturated fat 6 g; Protein 59.9 g; Carbohydrate 71 g; Fibre 6.1 g; Cholesterol 217 mg

WILD RICE AND MIXED MUSHROOM PILAF

THIS EASY RECIPE CAN BE SERVED AS A VEGETARIAN MAIN MEAL OR SIDE DISH. FOR AN EVEN LOWER GI VERSION, YOU CAN SUBSTITUTE THE WILD RICE WITH COARSE BURGHUL.

125 g (4½ oz/⅔ cup) wild rice
375 ml (13 fl oz/1½ cups) salt-reduced
  vegetable stock
1½ tbsp reduced-fat olive or canola oil
  margarine
1 large onion, finely chopped
2 garlic cloves, crushed
250 g (9 oz/1¼ cups) basmati rice
300 g (10½ oz) mixed mushrooms, sliced
1½ tbsp chopped thyme
1 fresh bay leaf

300 g (10½ oz) tinned chickpeas, rinsed
  and drained
60 g (2¼ oz) baby spinach leaves
2 tbsp chopped flat-leaf (Italian) parsley
2 tbsp pine nuts, lightly toasted, to serve

PREP TIME: 20 MINUTES + 5 MINUTES
  STANDING
COOKING TIME: 50 MINUTES
SERVES 4–6

Rinse the wild rice and cook in a saucepan of plenty of boiling water for 25 minutes—it will only be partially cooked after this time. Drain.

When the rice is nearly done, pour the stock into a large saucepan with 375 ml (13 fl oz/1½ cups) water and bring to the boil. Reduce the heat to a simmer.

Meanwhile, melt the margarine in a large frying pan. Add the onion and garlic and cook for 3–4 minutes, or until the onion is softened but not browned. Add the basmati rice and stir until the rice grains are coated with margarine, then stir in the mushrooms.

Add the wild rice, stock, thyme and bay leaf. Bring to the boil while stirring, then reduce the heat, cover tightly with a lid and simmer for 15 minutes, or until the rice is tender and the stock has been absorbed.

Leave to stand for 5 minutes. Remove the bay leaf. Season with freshly ground black pepper, add the chickpeas, spinach leaves and parsley and fluff up the rice with a fork until well mixed and the spinach has wilted. Sprinkle with pine nuts and serve.

HINT:
• Try a mix of button, field and Swiss brown mushrooms.

nutrition per serve (6): Energy 2117 kJ (506 Cal); Fat 13.3 g; Saturated fat 1.5 g; Protein 14.8 g; Carbohydrate 77 g; Fibre 9.3 g; Cholesterol 0 mg

SPICY CHICKEN BURGERS

500 g (1 lb 2 oz) lean minced (ground)
  chicken
4 spring onions (scallions), finely chopped
4 tbsp finely chopped coriander (cilantro)
  leaves
2 garlic cloves, crushed
¼ tsp cayenne pepper
1 egg white, lightly beaten
1 tbsp olive or canola oil

1 lemon, halved
150 g (5½ oz) tabouleh
  (see recipe on page 95)
4 wholegrain bread rolls, halved (see Hint)

PREP TIME: 10 MINUTES + 20 MINUTES
  REFRIGERATION
COOKING TIME: 10 MINUTES
SERVES 4

Mix together the chicken, spring onion, coriander, garlic, cayenne pepper and egg white and season with a little salt and freshly ground black pepper. Shape the mixture into four patties. Refrigerate for 20 minutes before cooking.

Heat the oil in a large non-stick frying pan over medium heat, add the patties and cook for about 5 minutes on each side, or until browned and cooked through.

Squeeze the lemon on the cooked patties and drain well on paper towels. Add the patties to the halved wholegrain buns and fill with the tabouleh.

HINT:
• The coarser the bread, the lower the GI.

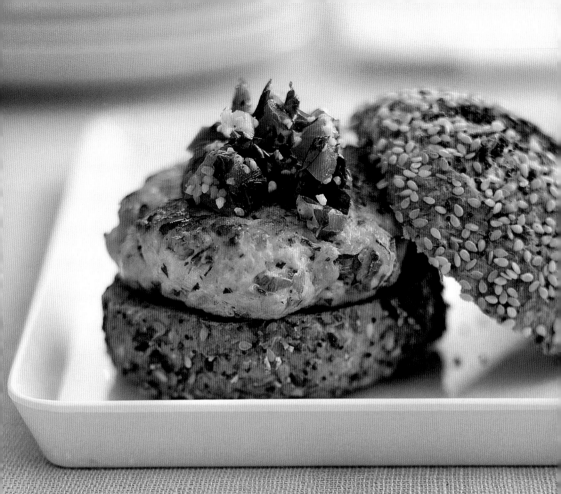

THESE CHICKEN BURGERS ARE
EASY TO MAKE AND ARE A MUCH
HEALTHIER ALTERNATIVE TO
REGULAR TAKE-AWAY BURGERS.

nutrition per serve: Energy 1615 kJ (386 Cal)
Fat 14.1 g
Saturated fat 2.5 g
Protein 20.4 g
Carbohydrate 40.4 g
Fibre 6.6 g
Cholesterol 98 mg

SWEET THINGS

STRAWBERRY AND BANANA ICE

THIS DESSERT IS A DELICIOUS ALTERNATIVE TO ICE CREAM AND SUITABLE FOR PEOPLE WHO ARE INTOLERANT TO DAIRY FOODS. IT PROVIDES ANTIOXIDANTS, FIBRE AND MOST MINERALS.

300 g (10½ oz) silken tofu, chopped
250 g (9 oz/1⅓ cups) strawberries, roughly chopped
2 just-ripe bananas, roughly chopped
7 g (⅛ oz/¼ cup) sucralose or 55 g (2 oz/ ¼ cup) caster (superfine) sugar (see Hints)

PREP TIME: 15 MINUTES + FREEZING
COOKING TIME: NIL
SERVES 4

Place the tofu, strawberries, bananas and sucralose or caster sugar in a blender or food processor and process until smooth.

Pour the mixture into a shallow cake tin and freeze for 3 hours, or until almost frozen. Break up roughly with a fork or a spoon, then transfer to a large bowl and beat until it has a smooth texture. Pour the mixture evenly into a suitable container, cover and freeze again, until quite firm.

Alternatively, freeze the blended mixture in an ice cream machine according to the manufacturer's instructions, until thick and creamy, then store in a covered container in the freezer.

Transfer to the refrigerator for about 30 minutes before serving to allow the ice to soften slightly. Scoop the ice into bowls to serve.

HINTS:
• Silken tofu is readily available in the refrigerated section of most supermarkets and health food shops. You can also buy it in long-life packets. Make sure you buy silken tofu as this type does not go lumpy.
• Many dietitians advise diabetics to use sucralose instead of sugar when cooking. The nutritional information below has been assessed using sucralose.
• If you use caster sugar instead of sucralose, the dessert will contain more calories and have a slightly higher GI. However, it will still remain in the low-GI range.

nutrition per serve: Energy 643 kJ (154 Cal); Fat 5.2 g; Saturated fat 0.7 g; Protein 10.8 g; Carbohydrate 14.2 g; Fibre 3.8 g; Cholesterol 0 mg

FROZEN FRUIT YOGHURT

THIS SWEET TREAT IS A GOOD SOURCE OF CALCIUM AND FIBRE AND IS NICE AS A DESSERT OR SNACK—TRY FREEZING SOME INTO ICEBLOCK (POPSICLE/ ICE LOLLY) MOULDS FOR HEALTHY TREATS ON HOT DAYS.

205 g (7¼ oz/1 cup) chopped mixed low-GI fresh fruit (apple, just-ripe banana, peach, apricot, orange)
250 g (9 oz/1 cup) low-fat plain unsweetened yoghurt

PREP TIME: 5 MINUTES + 4 HOURS FREEZING
COOKING TIME: NIL
SERVES 4

Put the mixed fruit in a blender, add the yoghurt and purée. Pour the mixture into a freezer tray and freeze.

For a lighter texture, remove the mixture from the freezer, return to the blender and whip, then refreeze. Repeat once more.

HINTS:
• Serve with a low-GI fruit salad: apples, pears, plums, nectarines, peaches, strawberries, just-ripe banana, mango, citrus fruit.
• The nutrition will vary depending on the type/ratio of fruit used.

nutrition per serve: Energy 239 kJ (57 Cal); Fat 0.2 g; Saturated fat 0.7 g; Protein 4.2 g; Carbohydrate 8.5 g; Fibre 1 g; Cholesterol 3 mg

THIS LOW-FAT, LOW-GI
DESSERT IS LIGHT AND EASY
TO MAKE. IT IS A NICE
ALTERNATIVE TO ICE CREAM OR
PUDDING AND IS PARTICULARLY
DELICIOUS DURING THE
SUMMER MONTHS.

nutrition per serve: Energy 705 kJ (168 Cal)
Fat 0.7 g
Saturated fat 0.3 g
Protein 18.1 g
Carbohydrate 17.9 g
Fibre 2.6 g
Cholesterol 10 mg

RASPBERRY MOUSSE

3 tsp powdered gelatine
250 g (9 oz/1 cup) low-fat vanilla yoghurt
with no added sugar
400 g (14 oz) light vanilla fromage frais
dessert
4 egg whites
150 g (5½ oz/1¼ cups) fresh raspberries,
coarsely mashed
fresh raspberries and mint leaves, to serve

PREP TIME: 30 MINUTES + CHILLING
COOKING TIME: NIL
SERVES 4–6

Sprinkle the gelatine over 1 tablespoon of water in a small heatproof bowl and leave to go spongy. Put the bowl in a saucepan of just boiled water, off the heat (the water should come halfway up the bowl). Stir until dissolved. Cool.

Combine the vanilla yoghurt and fromage frais dessert in a large bowl, then add the cooled gelatine and mix well.

Beat the egg whites until stiff peaks form, then fold through the yoghurt mixture until just combined. Transfer half the mixture to a separate bowl and fold in the mashed raspberries.

Divide the raspberry mixture among four tall glasses, then top with the vanilla mixture. Refrigerate for several hours, or until set. Decorate with extra fresh raspberries and mint leaves.

HINT:
• You can make this with frozen berries, but remember to thaw them before you use them.

MANGO PASSIONFRUIT SORBET

YOU CAN USE ANY COMBINATION OF FRUIT IN THIS RECIPE. THIS TANGY SORBET PROVIDES A REFRESHING BURST OF VITAMIN C AND A VARIETY OF ANTIOXIDANTS.

25 g (1 oz/1 cup) sucralose or 230 g
  (8½ oz/1 cup) caster sugar (see Hints)
90 g (3¼ oz/⅓ cup) passionfruit pulp
  (about 8 passionfruit)
½ large mango, chopped
1 large peach, chopped
2 tbsp lemon juice
1 egg white

PREP TIME: 20 MINUTES + 8 HOURS
  FREEZING
COOKING TIME: 5 MINUTES
SERVES 6

Put the sucralose in a saucepan with 250 ml (9 fl oz/1 cup) water. Stir over low heat until dissolved. Increase the heat, bring to the boil then transfer to a glass bowl, cool, then refrigerate. Strain the passionfruit pulp, reserving 1 tablespoon of the seeds.

Blend the fruit, passionfruit juice and lemon juice in a blender until smooth. With the motor running, add the cold sugar syrup and 150 ml (5 fl oz) water. Stir in the passionfruit seeds. Freeze in a shallow container, stirring occasionally, for about 2–3 hours without allowing it to become solid.

Break up the icy mixture roughly with a fork or spoon, transfer to a bowl and beat with electric beaters to combine. (It should remain icy.) Beat the egg white in a small bowl until firm peaks form, then fold into the mixture until just combined. Freeze for up to 1 hour or serve at once. It will solidify if frozen for longer.

HINTS:
• If you are making the sorbet with caster sugar, in Step 2, freeze the mixture for up to 5 hours. In Step 3, beat the mixture until smooth and fluffy. Beat the egg white in a small bowl until firm peaks form, then fold into the mixture until just combined. Spread into a loaf tin and return to the freezer until firm. Transfer to the refrigerator, to soften, 15 minutes before serving. The sorbet will contain more calories if you use sugar.
• To make a berry sorbet, use 200 g (7 oz) blackberries or blueberries, 200 g (7 oz) hulled strawberries and 50 g (1¾ oz) peach flesh. Prepare as above.

nutrition per serve: Energy 788 kJ (188 Cal); Fat 0.1 g; Saturated fat 0 g; Protein 1.6 g; Carbohydrate 44.7 g; Fibre 3 g; Cholesterol 0 mg

PEAR SORBET

THIS LOW-FAT, LOW-GI SORBET MAKES A REFRESHING DESSERT ON ITS OWN
OR YOU CAN SERVE IT WITH SOME CANNED PEARS AND LOW-FAT YOGHURT
OR ICE CREAM.

6 large (2 kg/4 lb 8 oz) very ripe pears
25 g (1 oz/1 cup) sucralose or 440 g
   (2 cups) sugar (see Hints)
200 ml (7 fl oz) water

PREP TIME: 40 MINUTES + OVERNIGHT
   FREEZING
COOKING TIME: 15 MINUTES
SERVES 4–6

Thickly peel the pears, then core them and slice them into thick pieces. Place the pears in a large saucepan, just cover with water and simmer for about 10 minutes, or until tender. Drain and set aside to cool.

Purée the pears in a blender or food processor until smooth.

Combine the sucralose and water in a saucepan over medium heat and stir through. After the sucralose has completely dissolved, take the syrup off the stove and set aside to cool.

Mix together the syrup and pear purée, then pour into a shallow metal pan. Freeze until just solid.

Remove the pan from the freezer. Beat or process until a 'slush' forms. Return to the pan and freeze until firm.

HINTS:
• Sorbets may be served before the main course to refresh the palate, or with other creams or fruit as a dessert.
• If you use sugar instead of sucralose the sorbet will contain more calories.

nutrition per serve: Energy 546 kJ (130 Cal); Fat 0.2 g; Saturated fat 0 g; Protein 0.6 g; Carbohydrate 30.8 g; Fibre 3.7 g; Cholesterol 0 mg

SUMMER FRUITY YOGHURT

2 ripe pears, unpeeled
2 tsp lemon juice
80 g (2¾ oz/½ cup) fresh or frozen
 blueberries
200 g (7 oz/1¼ cups) strawberries, hulled,
 halved and quartered
pulp of 2 passionfruit
1 tbsp sucralose or caster (superfine) sugar
 (see Hints)

500 g (1 lb 2 oz/2 cups) low-fat vanilla or
 fruit-flavoured yoghurt sweetened with
 a low-calorie sweetener
50 g (1¾ oz/⅓ cup) raw pistachio kernels,
 chopped

PREP TIME: 10 MINUTES + CHILLING TIME

COOKING TIME: NIL

SERVES 4

Remove the core from the pears. Cut into chunks and put into a large bowl, sprinkle with the lemon juice. Add the blueberries, strawberries and passionfruit and sprinkle with the sucralose or caster sugar. Set aside for 10 minutes to infuse. Gently fold through the yoghurt until just lightly coating the fruit.

Spoon into four 250 ml (9 fl oz/1 cup) parfait glasses and chill for at least 20 minutes. Sprinkle with the pistachios, to serve.

HINTS:
- For variety you can also make this recipe with raspberries, nectarines or peaches, or chopped citrus fruits.
- Using 1 tablespoon sugar instead of sucralose will increase the energy content and GI of this dessert, but it will still be low GI.
- Low-fat yoghurt that is sweetened with a low-calorie sweetener, instead of sugar, has less energy and a lower GI than sugar-sweetened low-fat yoghurt. Compare the sugar and energy values on yoghurt containers to find non-sugar sweetened varieties.

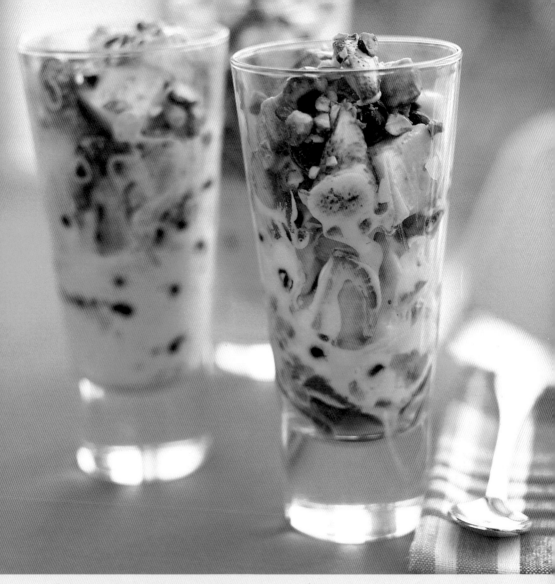

THIS LIGHT DESSERT IS GREAT IN
SUMMER, BUT IT CAN BE ENJOYED AT
ANY TIME OF YEAR USING THE LOW-GI
FRUIT THAT'S IN SEASON. IT TAKES
LITTLE TIME TO PREPARE AND IS
STYLISH ENOUGH TO SERVE AT A
CASUAL DINNER PARTY.

nutrition per serve: Energy 893 kJ (213 Cal)

Fat 6.8 g

Saturated fat 0.8 g

Protein 11.1 g

Carbohydrate 23.6 g

Fibre 5.7 g

Cholesterol 10 mg

FRUIT JELLIES

THESE LOW-GI HOME-MADE FRUIT JELLIES CONTAIN NO ARTIFICIAL COLOURS OR FLAVOURS. THE BERRIES PROVIDE SOME FIBRE, FOLATE AND ANTIOXIDANTS.

4 tsp gelatine
500 ml (17 fl oz/2 cups) cranberry and
   raspberry juice
330 g (11¾ oz) mixed berries, fresh or
   frozen

PREP TIME: 20 MINUTES + REFRIGERATION
COOKING TIME: NIL
SERVES 4

Sprinkle the gelatine in an even layer onto 3 tablespoons of the juice, in a small bowl, and leave to go spongy. Bring a small pan of water to the boil, remove from the heat and place the bowl in the pan. The water should come halfway up the side of the bowl. Stir the gelatine until clear and dissolved. Cool slightly and mix with the rest of the juice.

Rinse four 185 ml (6 fl oz/¾ cup) moulds with water (wet moulds make it easier when unmoulding) and pour 2 cm of the juice into each. Refrigerate until set.

Meanwhile, if the fruit is frozen, defrost it and add any liquid to the remaining juice. When the bottom layer of jelly has set, divide the fruit among the moulds (reserving a few berries to garnish) and divide the rest of the juice among the moulds, pouring it over the fruit. Refrigerate until set.

To turn out the jellies, hold each mould in a hot, damp tea towel and turn out onto a plate. Ease away the edge of the jelly with your finger to break the seal. (If you turn the jellies onto a damp plate you will be able to move them around, otherwise they will stick.) Garnish with the reserved berries.

nutrition per serve: Energy 353 kJ (84 Cal); Fat 0.1 g; Saturated fat 0 g; Protein 4.3 g; Carbohydrate 15.5 g; Fibre 1.9 g; Cholesterol 0 mg

SPICED POACHED PEARS

ENJOY THE DELICATE FLAVOURS OF THIS LOW-FAT DESSERT. THE PEARS ARE EASILY DIGESTED AND PROVIDE POTASSIUM AND SOLUBLE FIBRE. SERVE THEM WITH YOGHURT FOR EXTRA PROTEIN, CALCIUM AND PHOSPHORUS.

6 beurre bosc pears
300 ml (10½ fl oz) rosé wine (see Hint)
150 ml (5 fl oz) pure apple or pear juice
4 cloves
1 vanilla bean, halved
1 cinnamon stick
1 tbsp pure maple syrup

200 g (7 oz) low-fat vanilla yoghurt
 sweetened with a low-calorie sweetener

PREP TIME: 10 MINUTES + 30 MINUTES
 STANDING
COOKING TIME: 20 MINUTES
SERVES 6

Peel, halve and core the pears. Place in a deep frying pan with a lid, and add the wine or water, fruit juice and cloves. Scrape the seeds out of the vanilla bean and add both the seeds and pod to the pan. Stir in the cinnamon stick and maple syrup. Bring to the boil, then reduce the heat and simmer for 5–7 minutes, or until the pears are tender. Remove from the heat and cover with the lid.

Leave the fruit for 30 minutes to allow the flavours to infuse, then remove the pears with a slotted spoon and place in a serving dish. Return the syrup to the heat and boil for 6–8 minutes, or until reduced by half. Strain the syrup over the pears. Serve warm or chilled with the yoghurt.

HINT:
• If you'd prefer not to use wine, the same amount of liquid can be replaced with additional apple and pear juice.

nutrition per serve: Energy 728 kJ (174 Cal); Fat 0.3 g; Saturated fat 0.04 g; Protein 2.5 g; Carbohydrate 32.4 g; Fibre 3.4 g; Cholesterol 3 mg

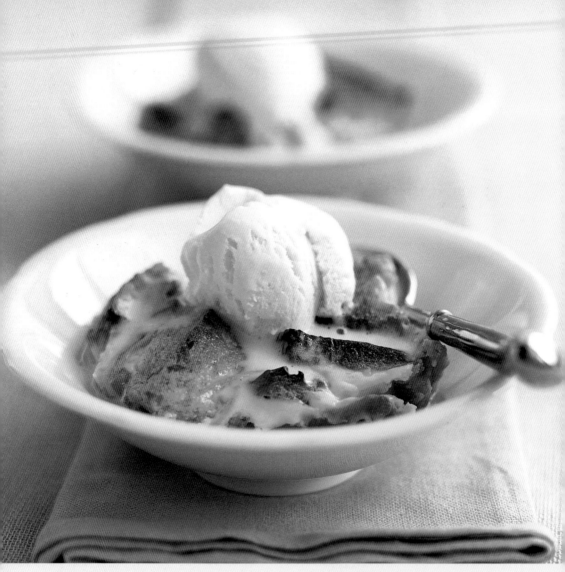

THIS NEW VERSION OF BREAD AND
BUTTER PUDDING HAS LESS FAT AND
BREAD AND MORE CUSTARD THAN
USUAL, GIVING THE PUDDING A SOFTER
TEXTURE. IT IS A GREAT WINTER
DESSERT BUT IT ISN'T LOW IN
CALORIES—SO ENJOY IN MODERATION.

nutrition per serve: Energy 709 kJ (169 Cal)

Fat 3.1 g

Saturated fat 0.8 g

Protein 8.9 g

Carbohydrate 25.2 g

Fibre 3.2 g

Cholesterol 65 mg

BAKED FRUIT BREAD CUSTARD

4 slices low-GI wholegrain fruit bread

1 tbsp sugar-free marmalade spread

80 g (2¾ oz/½ cup) chopped dried peaches

2 eggs

1 egg white

7 g (⅛ oz/¼ cup) sucralose or 55 g (2 oz/
 ¼ cup) caster (superfine) sugar (see Hints)

1 tsp grated lemon zest

500 ml (17 fl oz/2 cups) low-fat milk

freshly grated nutmeg, to sprinkle

PREP TIME: 15 MINUTES

COOKING TIME: 35 MINUTES

SERVES 6

Preheat the oven to 170°C (325°C/Gas 3). Spread the bread slices with the marmalade spread, cut each bread slice into quarters and arrange in a 1.25 litre (44 fl oz/5 cup) ceramic baking dish. Scatter with the chopped peaches.

Whisk together the eggs, egg white, sucralose or caster sugar and lemon zest in a bowl. Whisk in the milk. Pour over the bread and sprinkle with nutmeg. Set aside for 5 minutes to allow the bread to soften.

Put the dish in a roasting tin of hot water. The water should come halfway up the sides of the dish. Bake for 35 minutes, or until set. Serve with low-fat ice cream or low-fat yoghurt.

HINTS:
- If you use sugar instead of sucralose, the dessert will contain more calories and have a slightly higher GI. However, it will still remain in the low-GI range.
- There are many different types of fruit bread on the market and not all of them are low GI so you will need to read the label carefully.

DRIED APRICOT FOOL

THIS LOW-FAT FRUIT DESSERT IS RICH IN POTASSIUM AND BETACAROTENE. IT IS A GOOD SOURCE OF FIBRE AND PROVIDES A LITTLE IRON. IT SHOULD ONLY BE AN OCCASIONAL TREAT THOUGH AS IT IS NOT LOW IN CALORIES.

30 g (1 oz) finely chopped glacé ginger
175 g (6 oz) dried apricots, chopped
2 egg whites
2 tbsp sucralose or 2 tbsp caster (superfine) sugar

1 tbsp shredded coconut, toasted

PREP TIME: 15 MINUTES
COOKING TIME: 5 MINUTES
SERVES 4

Place the ginger, apricots and 4 tablespoons water in a small saucepan. Cook, covered, over a very low heat for 5 minutes, stirring occasionally. Remove from the heat and allow to cool completely.

Using electric beaters, beat the egg whites in a clean, dry bowl until soft peaks form. Add the sucralose or caster sugar and beat until just combined. Quickly and gently fold the cooled apricot mixture into the egg mixture and divide among four chilled serving glasses. Scatter the toasted coconut over the top and serve immediately.

HINTS:
• When adding the sucralose, be sure not to beat it for too long as it can clump and be difficult to fold.
• The apricots can scorch easily, so cook over low heat. Serve immediately, or the egg white will slowly break down and lose volume.
• If you use caster sugar instead of sucralose, the dessert will contain more calories and have a slightly higher GI. However, it will still remain in the low-GI range.

nutrition per serve: Energy 570 kJ (136 Cal); Fat 1.1 g; Saturated fat 0.9 g; Protein 3.7 g; Carbohydrate 26.1 g; Fibre 4.3 g; Cholesterol 0 mg

STONE-FRUIT SALAD

A COLOURFUL, REFRESHING DESSERT, BASED ON LOW-GI FRUIT, THAT'S QUICK AND EASY TO MAKE, AND A RICH SOURCE OF ANTIOXIDANTS.

4 apricots, unpeeled, halved and thinly sliced

4 peaches, unpeeled, halved and thinly sliced

4 nectarines, unpeeled, halved and thinly sliced

4 plums, unpeeled, halved and thinly sliced

2 tbsp unsweetened apricot juice or nectar

200 g (7 oz) light vanilla fromage frais dessert

PREP TIME: 15 MINUTES

COOKING TIME: NIL

SERVES 4

Mix the fruit together and drizzle with apricot juice. Serve the fruit salad with the fromage frais dessert.

HINT:
• You can replace the fromage frais dessert with low-fat ice cream or yoghurt, if you prefer.

nutrition per serve: Energy 881 kJ (211 Cal); Fat 0.7 g; Saturated fat 0.1 g; Protein 8 g; Carbohydrate 36.3 g; Fibre 8.2 g; Cholesterol 3 mg

APPLE AND STRAWBERRY CRUMBLE

800 g (1 lb 12 oz) tinned unsweetened apple pie fruit
250 g (9 oz/1⅔ cups) strawberries, hulled and sliced
75 g (2¾ oz/¾ cup) wholegrain rolled oats
7 g (⅛ oz/¼ cup) sucralose or 55 g (2 oz/ ¼ cup) soft brown sugar (see Hint)
50 g (1¾ oz/¼ cup) stoneground wholemeal (wholewheat) plain (all-purpose) flour

1 tbsp pepitas (pumpkin seeds)
1½ tbsp cold reduced-fat olive or canola oil margarine
low-fat, sugar-free vanilla or strawberry yoghurt, to serve

PREP TIME: 10 MINUTES
COOKING TIME: 20 MINUTES
SERVES 6

Preheat the oven to 180°C (350°F/Gas 4). Place the apples in a 1.5-litre (52 fl oz/6 cup), deep 20 x 5 cm (8 x 2 in) ovenproof dish. Stir through the strawberries.

Combine the rolled oats, sucralose or brown sugar, flour and pepitas in a bowl. Rub in the margarine, using the fingertips, until crumbly. Do not overmix. Spread evenly over the apple. Bake for 20 minutes, or until golden brown. Serve with the yoghurt.

HINT:
• If you use brown sugar instead of sucralose, the dessert will contain more calories and have a slightly higher GI. However, it will still remain in the low-GI range.

THIS DESSERT DELIVERS
EVERYTHING YOU WANT IN A
CRUMBLE WITH LESS FAT AND
CALORIES THAN TRADITIONAL
FRUIT CRUMBLES.

nutrition per serve: Energy 799 kJ (191 Cal)

Fat 5.3 g

Saturated fat 1.7 g

Protein 3.8 g

Carbohydrate 30 g

Fibre 4.9

Cholesterol 0 mg

ORANGE SEMOLINA CAKE

EVERYONE NEEDS SOMETHING SWEET NOW AND THEN AND THIS CAKE IS A
GREAT CHOICE FOR AN OCCASIONAL TREAT. IT IS LOW GI, BUT IT IS STILL
A HIGH CALORIE TREAT, SO ENJOY IN MODERATION.

olive or canola oil spray
150 g (5½ oz/1 cup) stoneground self-
raising flour
125 g (4½ oz/1 cup) semolina
55 g (2 oz/½ cup) ground almonds
10 g (¼ oz/⅓ cup) sucralose or 80 g
(2½ oz/⅓ cup) raw sugar (see Hints)
3 eggs
3 tbsp reduced-fat olive or canola oil
margarine, just melted
250 ml (9 fl oz/1 cup) buttermilk

2 tbsp orange juice
1 tbsp grated orange zest

PREP TIME: 20 MINUTES
COOKING TIME: 50 MINUTES
SERVES 8–10

Preheat the oven to 170°C (325°F/Gas 3). Lightly spray a 20 cm (8 in) round cake tin with
oil, then line the base with baking paper.

Sift the flour into a large bowl, add the semolina, ground almonds and sucralose, then
return any husks to the bowl. Mix together and make a well in the centre.

Put the eggs, margarine, buttermilk, orange juice and orange zest in a bowl and whisk until
well combined. Stir into the flour mixture and mix until smooth. Spoon into the prepared
tin and smooth the surface.

Bake for 45–50 minutes, or until cooked when tested with a metal skewer. Leave in the tin
for 10 minutes, then turn out onto a wire rack to cool completely (you may need to gently
loosen the cake from the tin with a knife). Serve in wedges with some berries, stone fruit
or orange slices and low-fat yoghurt.

HINTS:
• The cake will keep refrigerated for up to 1 week. Freeze for up to 1 month.
• If you are using raw sugar, this will raise the cake's GI into the medium-GI range. It will
also contain more calories.

nutrition per serve (10): Energy 788 kJ (188 Cal); Fat 7.8 g; Saturated fat 1.4 g; Protein 6.9 g;
Carbohydrate 21.7 g; Fibre 1.5 g; Cholesterol 59 mg

FRUITY LAYER CAKE

THIS DELICIOUS, MOIST CAKE CONTAINS FEWER CALORIES THAN TRADITIONAL FRUIT CAKE AND IS STYLISH ENOUGH TO SERVE AT A SPECIAL OCCASION OR BAKE AS A GIFT FOR A FRIEND. ALTHOUGH LOW GI, THIS CAKE IS ENERGY-DENSE SO ENJOY ONE SLICE AS AN OCCASIONAL TREAT.

1 large green apple, peeled, cored and chopped

90 g (3¼ oz/⅓ cup) chopped pitted prunes

60 g (2¼ oz/⅓ cup) chopped dried apricots

60 g (2¼ oz/⅓ cup) chopped dried peaches or dried pears

½ tsp ground cinnamon

olive or canola oil spray

3 tbsp reduced-fat olive or canola oil margarine

14 g (½ oz/½ cup) sucralose or 115 g (4 oz/½ cup) soft brown sugar

2 eggs

200 g (7 oz/1⅓ cups) stoneground wholemeal self-raising flour

25 g (1 oz/¼ cup) desiccated coconut

2 tbsp unprocessed oat bran

185 ml (6 oz/¾ cup) low-fat milk

PREP TIME: 25 MINUTES

COOKING TIME: 1 HOUR

SERVES 10–12

To make the filling, put the chopped apple, prunes, apricots and peaches and cinnamon in a saucepan with 125 ml (4 fl oz/½ cup) water. Cover and cook over low heat for 10–15 minutes, or until the fruit has softened and the water has been absorbed. Cool.

Preheat the oven to 180°C (350°F/Gas 4). Spray a deep 20 cm (8 in) square cake tin with oil, then line the base with baking paper.

To make the cake batter, put the margarine and sucralose or brown sugar in a bowl and beat with electric beaters for 1 minute. Add the eggs one at a time, beating well after each addition. (If using the sucralose the mixture will look curdled.)

Fold the combined sifted flour, including any husks, coconut and oat bran into the batter alternating with the milk. Spread half the batter over the base of the prepared tin. Spoon over the cooled fruit and roughly spoon the remaining batter over the fruit. There will be gaps of fruit showing.

Bake for 45 minutes, or until a skewer inserted in the centre comes out clean, and the cake is lightly golden brown on top. Cool in the tin for 10 minutes, then turn out onto a wire rack to cool. Serve warm or cold.

nutrition per serve (12): Energy 648 kJ (155 Cal); Fat 4.7 g; Saturated fat 1.9 g; Protein 4.8 g; Carbohydrate 21.4 g; Fibre 4.1 g; Cholesterol 32 mg

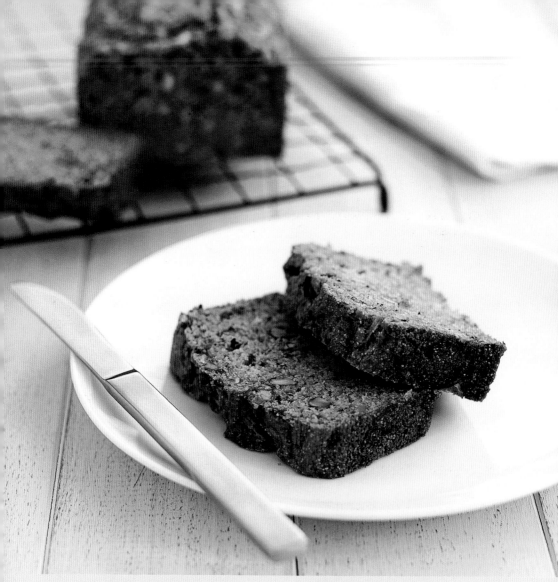

THIS SWEET BREAD HAS A
DELICIOUS FLAVOUR COMBINATION
THAT IS GREAT AT ANY TIME OF
DAY. YOU CAN FREEZE INDIVIDUAL
SLICES OF THIS LOAF TO PACK INTO
LUNCHBOXES OR PICNIC HAMPERS.

nutrition per serve: Energy 824 kJ (197 Cal)
Fat 10.7 g
Saturated fat 1.2 g
Protein 4.6 g
Carbohydrate 20 g
Fibre 1.7 g
Cholesterol 31 mg

ZUCCHINI AND PISTACHIO LOAF

olive or canola oil spray

150 g (5½ oz/1 cup) stoneground self-
raising flour

½ tsp freshly grated nutmeg

½ tsp bicarbonate of soda (baking soda)

90 g (3¼ oz/¾ cup) semolina

50 g (1¾ oz/1⁄4 cup) soft brown sugar (or
half sucralose, see Hints)

80 g (2¾ oz/½ cup) raw pistachio nuts,
chopped

2 eggs

90 g (3¼ oz/⅓ cup) unsweetened apple
purée

4 tbs olive or canola oil

2 tsp grated lemon or lime zest

140 g (5 oz/1 cup) grated zucchini
(courgette)

PREP TIME: 20 MINUTES

COOKING TIME: 50 MINUTES

MAKES 10–12 SLICES

Preheat the oven to 170°C (325°F/Gas 3). Spray a 19.5 x 9.5 cm (7½ x 3¾ in) loaf tin with oil, then line the base with baking paper.

Sift the flour, nutmeg and bicarbonate of soda into a large bowl, then return any husks to the bowl. Stir in the semolina, brown sugar and pistachio nuts. Make a well in the centre.

Whisk together the eggs, apple purée, oil and lemon zest in a bowl. Squeeze out any excess moisture from the grated zucchini, then stir into the egg mixture. Add all at once to the flour mixture and stir until combined and smooth. Spoon into the prepared tin and smooth the surface.

Bake for 45–50 minutes, or until cooked when tested with a metal skewer. Leave in the tin for 10 minutes, then turn out onto a wire rack to cool completely. Cut into slices to serve.

HINTS:
• You can replace half the sugar with sucralose if you prefer. The sucralose will lower the GI and calorie content of the loaf, which is good if you have diabetes or are watching your weight.
• You will need 2 medium zucchini (courgettes) to yield 1 cup grated.
• The loaf will keep refrigerated for up to 1 week and can be stored frozen for up to 1 month.

MIXED FRUIT AND BANANA BREAD

THE DRIED FRUIT IN THIS NEW VERSION OF BANANA BREAD PACKS A LOT OF FLAVOUR INTO EACH SLICE. THIS LOW-GI BREAD IS MORE NUTRITIOUS THAN MANY CAKES AND BISCUITS, BUT SHOULD STILL BE ENJOYED IN MODERATION AS AN OCCASSIONAL TREAT.

olive or canola oil spray
250 g (9 oz/1⅔ cups) stoneground
   self-raising flour
1 tsp baking powder
1 tsp mixed spice
100 g (3½ oz) chopped dried pears
100 g (3½ oz) chopped dried peaches
35 g (1¼ oz/¼ cup) natural oat bran
9 g (¾ oz/⅓ cup) sucralose or 80 g
   (2¾ oz/⅓ cup) caster (superfine) sugar
   (see Hints)

70 g (2½ oz/½ cup) hazelnuts, roughly
   chopped (optional)
2 eggs
310 g (11 oz/1¼ cups) plain low-fat yoghurt
3 tbsp canola oil
1 large just-ripe banana, mashed

PREP TIME: 20 MINUTES

COOKING TIME: 50 MINUTES

MAKES 10–12 SLICES

Preheat the oven to 170°C (325°F/Gas 3). Spray a 22 x 14 cm (8½ x 5½ in) loaf tin with oil, then line the base with baking paper.

Sift the flour, baking powder and mixed spice into a large bowl, then return any husks to the bowl. Stir in the dried pears and peaches and use your hands to mix and separate the chopped fruit. Stir in the oat bran, sucralose or caster sugar and chopped hazelnuts.

Whisk together the eggs, yoghurt, oil and mashed banana in a bowl. Add to the flour mixture and stir until combined and smooth. Spoon into the prepared tin and smooth the surface.

Bake for 50 minutes, or until a skewer inserted in the centre comes out clean. Cover with foil for the last 10 minutes if it is browning too much. Leave in the tin for 15 minutes, then turn out onto a wire rack to cool. Cut into slices to serve. Serve warm or cold. Delicious toasted.

HINTS:
• Using caster sugar instead of sucralose will increase the bread's GI and calorie content, but the bread will remain in the low-GI range.
• Will keep refrigerated for up to 1 week. Freeze for up to 1 month.
• Eat it as a treat only as the hazelnuts are quite high in fat. If preferred, you can leave them out.

nutrition per serve (12): Energy 992 kJ (237 Cal); Fat 9.6 g; Saturated fat 0.8 g; Protein 6.7 g; Carbohydrate 29.1 g; Fibre 3.6 g; Cholesterol 33 mg

CARROT WALNUT LOAF

THIS IS A HEALTHIER CHOICE THAN COMMERCIAL CARROT CAKE OR
CHOCOLATE CAKE BUT IT'S NOT LOW IN CALORIES.

olive or canola oil spray
150 g (5½ oz/1 cup) stoneground self-
   raising flour
½ tsp bicarbonate of soda (baking soda)
1 tsp ground cinnamon
90 g (3¼ oz/¾ cup) coarse semolina
9 g (¾ oz/⅓ cup) sucralose or 80 g
   (2¾ oz/⅓ cup) raw sugar (see Hints)
60 g (2¼ oz/½ cup) walnuts, chopped
60 g (2¼ oz/½ cup) dried-fruit medley

235 g (8½ oz/1½ cups) grated carrot
2 eggs
250 ml (9 fl oz/1 cup) buttermilk
4 tbsp olive or canola oil

PREP TIME: 20 MINUTES
COOKING TIME: 50 MINUTES
MAKES 10–12 SLICES

Preheat the oven to 170°C (325°F/Gas 3). Spray a 19.5 x 9.5 cm (7½ in x 3¾ in) loaf tin
with oil, then line the base with baking paper.

Sift the flour, bicarbonate of soda and cinnamon into a large bowl, then return any husks to
the bowl. Stir in the semolina and sucralose or raw sugar, then stir in the walnuts, fruit
medley and grated carrot. Make a well in the centre.

Whisk together the eggs, buttermilk and oil in a bowl. Add to the flour mixture and stir
until combined and smooth. Spoon into the prepared tin and smooth the surface.

Bake for 50 minutes, or until a skewer inserted in the centre comes out clean. Leave in
the tin for 10 minutes, then turn out onto a wire rack to cool completely. Cut into slices
to serve.

HINTS:
- Using raw sugar instead of sucralose will increase the loaf's GI and calorie content, but
  the loaf will remain in the low-GI range.
- Will keep refrigerated for up to 1 week and frozen for up to 1 month.
- Fruit medley is a mixture of dried apple, apricots, pears and sultanas.

nutrition per serve (12): Energy 851 kJ (203 Cal); Fat 11.1 g; Saturated fat 1.2 g; Protein 5 g;
Carbohydrate 19.8 g; Fibre 2.1 g; Cholesterol 33 mg

LEMON BERRY CHEESECAKE

FRUITY BASE
60 g (2¼ oz) dried apricots
60 g (2¼ oz) dried pitted dates
60 g (2¼ oz) dried figs
70 g (2½ oz/⅓ cup) coarse semolina

CHEESECAKE
300 g (10½ oz) low-fat ricotta cheese
2 tbsp sucralose or 2 tbsp caster sugar
  (see Hint)
250 g (9 oz) light French vanilla fromage
  frais

250 g (9 oz) low-fat lemon-flavoured
  fromage frais
2 tsp finely grated lemon zest
2 tbsp lemon juice
1 tbsp gelatine
2 egg whites
250 g (9 oz) strawberries, halved

PREP TIME: 25 MINUTES + OVERNIGHT
  REFRIGERATION
COOKING TIME: NIL
SERVES 12

Lightly oil and line the base and side of a 20 cm (8 in) spring-form cake tin with plastic wrap. Line the base, over the plastic, with baking paper. Process the dried fruit in a food processor until finely chopped; add the semolina and blend well together. Use fingers to spread evenly over the base of the prepared tin. Refrigerate.

Combine the ricotta and sucralose or sugar in a food processor until smooth. Add all the fromage frais, the lemon zest and juice, then mix well. Transfer to a large bowl.

Put 3 tablespoons of water in a small bowl, sprinkle the gelatine in an even layer onto the surface and leave to go spongy. Bring a small saucepan of water to the boil, remove from the heat and put the gelatine bowl in the pan. The water should come halfway up the side of the bowl. Stir the gelatine until clear and dissolved, then cool slightly. Stir the gelatine mixture into the ricotta mixture.

Beat the egg whites until soft peaks form, then gently fold into the ricotta mixture. Pour the mixture into the tin evenly over the fruity base and refrigerate for several hours or overnight, until set. Carefully remove from the tin by removing the side of the tin and easing the plastic from the sides. Use a spatula to aid in lifting the cheesecake off the baking paper, removing the plastic wrap. Put on a serving platter and decorate with the halved strawberries.

HINT:
• Using caster sugar instead of sucralose will increase the GI and calorie content, but the cheesecake will remain in the low-GI range.

THIS TANGY, LOW-FAT
CHEESECAKE PROVIDES
SOME BETACAROTENE,
CALCIUM AND PHOSPHORUS.

nutrition per serve: Energy 561 kJ (134 Cal)
Protein 8.8 g
Fat 1.5 g
Saturated fat 0.6 g
Carbohydrate 19.6 g
Fibre 2.3 g
Cholesterol 2 mg

WHOLEMEAL APRICOT ROCK CAKES

DELICIOUS SERVED WARM OR COLD, THESE CRUNCHY ROCK CAKES WILL QUICKLY BECOME A FAMILY FAVOURITE. THEY MAKE A NICE TREAT TO TAKE ALONG TO PICNICS.

225 g (8 oz/1½ cups) stoneground self-raising flour
1 tsp baking powder
1½ tsp ground cinnamon
25 g (1 oz/¼ cup) light dessicated coconut
35 g (1¼ oz/¼ cup) unprocessed oat bran
9 g (¾ oz/⅓ cup) sucralose or 80 g (2¾ oz/⅓ cup) raw sugar (see Hints)
3 tbsp cold reduced-fat olive or canola oil margarine

185 g (6½ oz/1 cup) dried apricots, chopped
1 tbsp sunflower or pepitas seeds
1 egg
4 tbsp low-fat milk

PREP TIME: 20 MINUTES
COOKING TIME: 20 MINUTES
MAKES 24

Preheat the oven to 180°C (350°F/Gas 4). Line a large baking tray with baking paper.

Sift the flour, baking powder and cinnamon into a large bowl, then return any husks to the bowl. Stir in the coconut, oat bran and sucralose or raw sugar. Using clean fingers, rub the margarine into the mixture until crumbly. Stir in the apricots and seeds. Make a well in the centre.

Combine the egg and milk in a small bowl. Pour into the well in the dry ingredients and mix briefly with a fork until just combined into a rough dough.

Using 1 heaped tablespoon of mixture at a time, put spoonfuls onto the tray, forming a little mound, then flatten slightly. Bake for 15–20 minutes, or until cooked and golden brown—watching carefully that they don't burn. Leave on the tray for 2–3 minutes then transfer to a wire rack to cool completely.

HINTS:
• Store in an airtight container for up to 5 days.
• Using sugar instead of sucralose will increase the rock cakes' GI and calorie content, but they will remain in the low-GI range.

nutrition per rock cake (24): Energy 339 kJ (81 Cal); Fat 2.6 g; Saturated fat 1.0 g; Protein 2.1 g; Carbohydrate 11.5 g; Fibre 1.6 g; Cholesterol 8 mg

HAZELNUT BROWNIES

KIDS AND ADULTS WILL LOVE THIS CRUNCHY TREAT, AND BEING SMALL THEY ARE EASY TO TAKE TO PICNICS, BARBECUES AND ON CAMPING TRIPS. FOR VARIETY AND EXTRA OMEGA-3 FAT, YOU CAN REPLACE THE HAZELNUTS WITH PECANS OR WALNUTS.

olive or canola oil spray

150 g (5½ oz/1 cup) stoneground
    self-raising flour

60 g (2¼ oz/½ cup) cocoa powder

½ teaspoon bicarbonate of soda
    (baking soda)

34 g (1¼ oz/1¼ cups) sucralose or 230 g
    (8½ oz/1¼ cups) raw sugar (see Hints)

60 g (2¼ oz/⅓ cup) dark chocolate chips

70 g (2½ oz/½ cup) raw hazelnuts, roughly
    chopped

2 eggs

250 ml (9 fl oz/1 cup) buttermilk

60 g (2¼ oz/¼ cup) unsweetened apple
    purée

2 tbsp olive or canola oil

1 tsp natural vanilla extract

icing (confectioners') sugar, to dust

PREP TIME: 15 MINUTES

COOKING TIME: 40 MINUTES

MAKES 14–16 SQUARES

Preheat the oven to 180°C (350°F/Gas 4). Spray a 27 x 17 cm (10¾ x 6½ in) shallow baking tin with oil, then line the base with baking paper overhanging the two long sides.

Sift the flour, cocoa and bicarbonate of soda into a large bowl, then return any husks to the bowl. Stir in the sucralose or raw sugar then the chocolate chips and hazelnuts. Make a well in the centre.

Whisk together the eggs, buttermilk, apple purée, oil and vanilla in a bowl. Add to the flour mixture and stir until just combined and smooth. Do not overmix. Pour into the prepared tin and smooth the surface.

Bake for 40 minutes, or until a skewer inserted in the centre comes out clean. Leave in the tin for 10 minutes, then turn out onto a wire rack to cool completely. Dust with icing sugar and cut into squares to serve.

HINTS:
• Store in an airtight container for up to 5 days.
• People with diabetes should make this recipe with sucralose rather than sugar because sugar will increase this recipe's calorie content and GI.

nutrition per square (16): Energy 598 kJ (143 Cal); Fat 7.6 g; Saturated fat 1.7 g; Protein 4 g; Carbohydrate 13.9 g; Fibre 1.1 g; Cholesterol 25 mg

THIS RECIPE IS QUICK AND EASY TO
MAKE AND IS SUITABLE FOR THE
WHOLE FAMILY AS A SPECIAL TREAT.
THE OATS MAKE THIS SLICE MORE
FILLING TO HELP YOU FEEL
SATISFIED WITH JUST ONE PIECE.

nutrition per serve (16): Energy 582 kJ (139 Cal)
Fat 7.3 g
Saturated fat 2 g
Protein 3.3 g
Carbohydrate 14.2 g
Fibre 2.3 g
Cholesterol 0.5 mg

CHOCOLATE FRUIT AND NUT SLICE

olive or canola oil spray

150 g (5½ oz/1 cup) stoneground wholemeal self-raising flour

2 tbsp unsweetened cocoa powder

50 g (1¾ oz/½ cup) wholegrain rolled oats

30 g (1 oz/⅓ cup) desiccated coconut

2 tbsp unprocessed oat bran

9 g (¾ oz/⅓ cup) sucralose or 60 g (2¼ oz/⅓ cup) soft brown sugar (see Hints)

60 g (2¼ oz/½ cup) dried-fruit medley, chopped

60 g (2¼ oz/½ cup) walnuts, chopped

90 g (3¼ oz) reduced-fat canola oil margarine, just melted

1 tbsp pure maple syrup

250 ml (9 fl oz/1 cup) low-fat milk

icing (confectioners') sugar, to dust

PREP TIME: 15 MINUTES

COOKING TIME: 25 MINUTES

MAKES 14–16 SLICES

Preheat the oven to 180°C (350°F/Gas 4). Spray a 27 x 17 cm (10¾ x 6½ in) shallow baking tin with oil, then line the base with baking paper overhanging the two long sides.

Sift the flour and cocoa into a large bowl, then return any husks to the bowl. Stir in the rolled oats, coconut, oat bran and sucralose or brown sugar, fruit medley and walnuts. Make a well in the centre.

Combine the melted margarine, maple syrup and milk in a small bowl. Add to the flour mixture and stir until well combined. Spread evenly into the prepared tin.

Bake for 25 minutes, or until cooked and firm. Leave in the tin to cool, then turn out onto a wire rack to cool completely. Dust with icing sugar and cut into slices to serve. Delicious served with berries and low-fat yoghurt or berry fromage frais.

HINTS:
- Will keep in an airtight container for 5 days. Freeze for up to 1 month.
- Replace walnuts with pecans if liked.
- If you have diabetes, this recipe is best made with sucralose or another low-calorie sugar substitute instead of sugar, because sugar will increase the slice's calorie content and effect on your blood sugar level.

GLUTEN-FREE PEAR MUFFINS

HOME-MADE MUFFINS LIKE THESE ARE EASY TO MAKE. FREE OF GLUTEN, NUTS AND SOY, THEY CAN ALSO BE MADE WITH OTHER FRUIT COMBINATIONS.

olive or canola oil, for greasing
250 g (9 oz/2 cups) soy-free, gluten-free
  self-raising flour
2 tsp gluten-free baking powder
21 g (¾ oz/¾ cup) sucralose or 140 g
  (5 oz/¾ cup) soft brown sugar (see Hints)
170 ml (5½ fl oz/⅔ cup) low-fat milk
4 tbsp olive or canola oil

2 eggs, or equivalent egg replacer
2 ripe pears (about 450 g/1 lb), peeled,
  cored and mashed

PREP TIME: 15 MINUTES
COOKING TIME: 20 MINUTES
MAKES 12

Preheat the oven to 180°C (350°F/Gas 4). Lightly grease a 12-hole muffin tin with oil.

Sift the flour and baking powder into a large bowl and add the sucralose or brown sugar. In a separate bowl, combine the milk, oil and eggs or egg replacer. Add the milk mixture and pears to the flour mixture. Use a large metal spoon to mix until just combined. Spoon the mixture into the muffin tin holes.

Bake for 18–20 minutes, or until a skewer inserted in the centre comes out clean. Leave for 5 minutes before turning onto a wire rack.

HINTS:
• These muffins need to be eaten the day they are made.
• Using sugar instead of sucralose will increase the muffins' GI and calorie content, but they will remain in the low- to medium-GI range.

nutrition per muffin: Energy 705 kJ (168 Cal); Fat 7.1 g; Saturated fat 0.7 g; Protein 2 g; Carbohydrate 24 g; Fibre 2.7 g; Cholesterol 32 mg

BERRY MUFFINS

THESE TANGY MUFFINS ARE PERFECT, SERVED WARM OR COLD, FOR
BREAKFAST, BRUNCH OR AFTERNOON TEA. THE BUTTERMILK ADDS FLAVOUR
AND LIGHTENS THE TEXTURE. THEY ARE NOT LOW IN CALORIES, SO ENJOY
IN MODERATION.

olive or canola oil spray
155 g (5½ oz/1¼ cups) stoneground
  self-raising flour
1 tsp baking powder
1 tsp ground cinnamon
35 g (1¼ oz/¼ cup) natural oat bran
50 g (1¾ oz/½ cup) wholegrain rolled oats
9 g (¾ oz/⅓ cup) sucralose or 80 g
  (2¾ oz/⅓ cup) caster (superfine) sugar
  (see Hints)
150 g (5½ oz/1 cup) blueberries, frozen or
  fresh

60 g (2¼ oz/½ cup) raspberries, frozen or
  fresh
1 egg
425 ml (15 fl oz) buttermilk
3 tbsp reduced-fat canola oil margarine,
  just melted
1 tsp natural vanilla extract
icing (confectioners') sugar, to dust

PREP TIME: 20 MINUTES

COOKING TIME: 25 MINUTES

MAKES 12

Preheat the oven to 180°C (350°F/Gas 4). Spray 12 x 80 ml (2½ fl oz/⅓ cup) muffin holes
with oil.

Sift the flour, baking powder and cinnamon into a large bowl, then return any husks to the
bowl. Stir in the oat bran, rolled oats, sucralose or caster sugar and berries. Make a well in
the centre.

Whisk together the egg, buttermilk, melted margarine and vanilla and stir into the flour
mixture until just combined. Do not overmix. Spoon evenly into the muffin holes.

Bake for 25 minutes, or until firm to touch. Leave in the tin for 5 minutes, then turn out
onto a wire rack to cool. Dust with icing sugar and serve warm or cold with fresh berries.

HINTS:
• Will keep refrigerated for up to 5 days or frozen for up to 1 month.
• These muffins can also be made in a mini muffin pan to produce small treats that can be
  added to a packed lunch.
• Using sugar instead of sucralose will increase the muffins' calorie content and GI value
  into the medium-GI category.

nutrition per muffin: Energy 615 kJ (147 Cal); Fat 4.4 g; Saturated fat 1.2 g; Protein 4.7 g;
Carbohydrate 20.6 g; Fibre 2 g; Cholesterol 19 mg

FRUIT AND OAT BRAN MUFFINS

olive or canola oil spray

225 g (8 oz/1½ cups) stoneground
　self-raising flour

1 tsp freshly grated nutmeg

½ tsp baking powder

150 g (5½ oz/1 cup) unprocessed oat bran

9 g (¾ oz/⅓ cup) sucralose or 80 g
　(2¾ oz/⅓ cup) raw sugar (see Hints)

125 g (4½ oz/1 cup) dried-fruit medley

1 egg

310 ml (11 fl oz/1¼ cups) low-fat milk

140 g (5 oz/½ cup) unsweetened apple
　purée

3 tbsp reduced-fat olive or canola oil
　margarine, just melted

PREP TIME: 20 MINUTES

COOKING TIME: 25 MINUTES

MAKES 12

Preheat the oven to 180°C (350°F/Gas 4). Spray 12 x 80 ml (2½ fl oz/⅓ cup) muffin holes with oil.

Sift the flour, nutmeg and the baking powder into a large bowl, then return any husks to the bowl. Stir in the oat bran, sucralose or raw sugar and fruit medley, using your fingertips to break up the fruit medley so it doesn't clump together. Make a well in the centre.

Whisk together the egg, milk, apple purée and melted margarine and stir into the flour mixture until just combined. Do not overmix. Spoon evenly into the muffin holes.

Bake for 25 minutes, or until firm to the touch and golden brown. Leave in the tin for 5 minutes, then turn out onto a wire rack to cool.

HINTS:
- If you use sugar instead of sucralose the muffins will contain more calories and be low- to medium-GI.
- To lower the GI further and add some healthy omega-3 fat, you can substitute 3 tablespoons of the flour with ground linseed (flaxseed) meal. This may reduce the cooking time a little, so check the muffins from 20 minutes onwards.
- Will keep refrigerated for up to 5 days and frozen for up to 1 month.

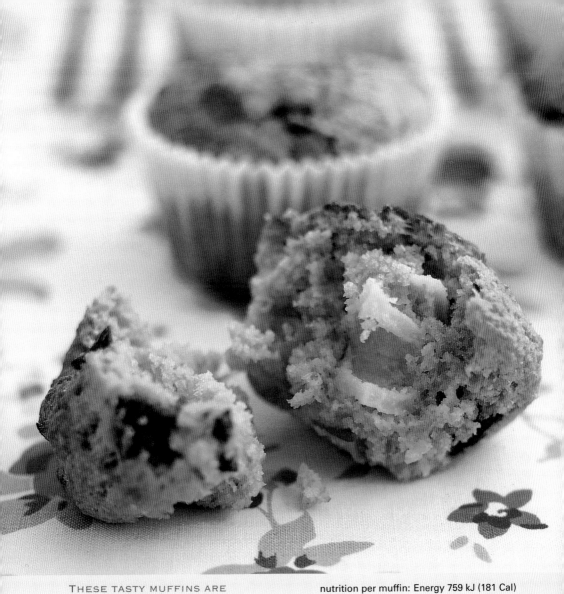

THESE TASTY MUFFINS ARE
A HEALTHY LOWER FAT
ALTERNATIVE TO COMMERCIAL
BRAN MUFFINS. HOWEVER,
THEY ARE NOT LOW IN
CALORIES, SO ENJOY
IN MODERATION.

nutrition per muffin: Energy 759 kJ (181 Cal)

Fat 4 g

Saturated fat 0.8 g

Protein 5.7 g

Carbohydrate 28.8 g

Fibre 3.6 g

Cholesterol 16 mg

Shopping list

bread

Bread and English muffins
with lots of grains in them
Pumpernickel bread (black
bread)
Sourdough bread—
wholegrain, rye, or
wholemeal
Fruit and spice loaf

breakfast cereals

Extruded bran cereals (not
bran flakes)
Semolina
Porridge made from
wholegrain traditional rolled
oats, steel-cut oats or rolled
barley (not instant or quick-
cooking oats)
Natural muesli with no or few
cereal flakes in it (based
on oats, nuts, seeds and
dried fruit)
Extruded rice bran

grains – for boiling – to be served with meals or added to soups and salads

Barley—pearled, pot
or cracked
Basmati rice
Doongara rice
Wild rice
Quinoa
Whole buckwheat kernels
Burghul (cracked wheat)
Whole rye kernels

pasta and noodles

All types of durum wheat
pasta—fresh or dried; plain,
wholemeal or protein-
enriched
Ravioli, tortellini
Gluten-free split pea and soy
pasta
Dried mung bean noodles
(lungkow beanthread or
cellophane)
Fresh rice noodles
(not dried)
Soba (buckwheat) noodles

biscuits/cookies

Biscuits that contain lots of
dried fruit, whole rolled oats,
and stoneground flour
Oatmeal biscuits

fruit

FRESH FRUIT
Apples, pears, oranges,
mandarins, tangerines,
grapefruit, plums, apricots,
nectarines, peaches, berries,
bananas (not over-ripe),
grapes, kiwi fruit, mango,
custard apple, chico,
avocado (high-fat—eat in
moderation)
DRIED FRUIT
Apple, apricot, pear, peach,
prunes, sultanas
CANNED FRUIT IN NATURAL
JUICE
peaches, pears

FRUIT JUICE — PURE,
UNSWEETENED, NO
ADDED SUGAR
Apple, grapefruit, orange,
pineapple, tomato

vegetables – fresh, canned and frozen

Butternut pumpkin and all-
purpose (waxy) potatoes—
not mashed
Green peas
Carrots, carrot juice
Sweet corn
All non-starchy, low-carb
vegetables – onions, garlic,
shallots, leeks, herbs,
rocket, ginger, chillies,
tomatoes, lettuce, celery,
cucumber, cabbage,
mushrooms, brussels
sprouts, broccoli,
cauliflower, capsicum,
spinach, green beans, snake
beans, kale, bean sprouts,
alfalfa, zucchini, eggplant,
artichokes, endive, chard,
silverbeet, bok choy and
other Asian greens, okra,
asparagus
Commercial tabouleh salad
(look for the least oily
looking ones)

legumes

All types of legumes—dried,
canned, vacuum packed
(e.g. lentils, chickpeas, soy

186

beans, kidney beans, cannellini beans, four bean mix)
Reduced-fat hummus dip
Tofu
Tempeh
Canned baked beans

nuts and seeds

All types of raw or dry-roasted nuts and seeds —eat in moderation (Use linseeds, ground linseed meal, walnuts and pecans in preference. These are relatively good sources of essential omega-3 fatty acids, which many people don't eat enough of.)

dairy products and some alternatives (fresh, frozen, long-life)

Cows' milk—full-fat, reduced-fat and low-fat; plain or flavoured
Soy milk, calcium-enriched—full-fat, reduced-fat, and low-fat
Fermented milk drinks
Yoghurt—all types
Custard
Ice cream—reduced and low-fat
Pudding—made from instant mix with milk
Mousse—made from instant

mix with milk or water; or reduced-fat varieties in chilled section of supermarket
Fromage frais products
All types of cheese—cottage, ricotta, reduced-fat cheddar and mozzarella

beverages

Bottled water—mineral, spring, soda
Diet soft drinks and diet cordials
Low-GI fruit juices (fresh in fridge or long-life)

sweeteners, condiments and other pantry staples

Sugar substitutes
Diet jams or pure fruit spreads with no added sugar
Yeast extract spreads
Low-fat mayonnaise and diet salad dressings
Vinegar, mustard, chilli sauce, mirin
Dried herbs and spices, capers, fresh herb mixes for fridge
Custard powder
Diet jelly crystals
Reduced-salt soy sauce
Canola and olive

oil, canola and olive oil spray, reduced-fat canola or olive oil margarine
Long-life lime juice and lemon juice
Grated parmesan cheese

meat, poultry, fish and seafood— fresh, frozen, canned

Lean cuts of meat and lower-fat premium mince
Poultry—fresh or frozen and eaten without the skin
Eggs
Low-fat deli meats and sausages
Fish—fresh or frozen; canned in spring water or flavoured in sachets
Seafood—fresh, frozen or canned
Sushi

soup—canned or dried

Minestrone
Lentil
Tomato
Clear beef, chicken or vegetable

CONTACT INFORMATION FOR DIABETES SUPPORT GROUPS

AUSTRALIA – Diabetes Australia
5th Floor, 39 London Circuit,
Canberra City, ACT 2600
Phone: 02 6232 3800
Email: admin@diabetesaustralia.com.au
Web: www.diabetesaustralia.com.au

INTERNATIONAL DIABETES INSTITUTE
250 Kooyong Road,
Caulfield, Victoria 3162
Phone: 03 9258 5050
Email: admin@idi.org.au
Web: www.diabetes.com.au

NEW ZEALAND – Diabetes New Zealand National Office
PO BOX 12-1441, Thorndon, Wellington
Phone: 04 499 7145
Email: info@diabetes.org.nz
Web: www.diabetes.org.nz

CANADA – Canadian Diabetes Association
National Life Building, 1400-522 University Ave
Toronto, ON M5G 2R5
Phone: 1 800 226 8464
Email:info@diabetes.ca
Web: www.diabetes.ca

UNITED KINGDOM– Diabetes UK
Macleod House,
10 Parkway, London NW1 7AA
Phone: 020 7424 1000
Email: info@diabetes.org.uk
Web: www.diabetes.org.uk

USA – American Diabetes Association
1701 North Beauregard Street,
Alexandria, VA 22311
Phone: 1 800 342 2383
Email: AskADA@diabetes.org
Web: www.diabetes.org

INDEX